Concepts of Evidence Based Practice for the Physical Therapist Assistant

Concepts *of* Evidence Based Practice *for the* Physical Therapist Assistant

Barbara B. Gresham, PT, PhD, GCS

Associate Professor and Director of the Doctor of Physical Therapy Program
University of Mary Hardin–Baylor
Belton, TX

 F.A. Davis Company • Philadelphia

F. A. Davis Company
1915 Arch Street
Philadelphia, PA 19103
www.fadavis.com

Printed in the United States of America

Last digit indicates print number: 10 9 8 7 6 5 4 3 2 1

Senior Acquisitions Editor: Melissa Duffield
Developmental Editor: Andrea Edwards
Director of Content Development: George Lang
Design and Illustration Manager: Carolyn O'Brien

As new scientific information becomes available through basic and clinical research, recommended treatments and drug therapies undergo changes. The author(s) and publisher have done everything possible to make this book accurate, up to date, and in accord with accepted standards at the time of publication. The author(s), editors, and publisher are not responsible for errors or omissions or for consequences from application of the book, and make no warranty, expressed or implied, in regard to the contents of the book. Any practice described in this book should be applied by the reader in accordance with professional standards of care used in regard to the unique circumstances that may apply in each situation. The reader is advised always to check product information (package inserts) for changes and new information regarding dose and contraindications before administering any drug. Caution is especially urged when using new or infrequently ordered drugs.

Library of Congress Cataloging-in-Publication Data

Gresham, Barbara B., author.
  Concepts of evidence-based practice for the physical therapist assistant / Barbara B. Gresham.
    p. ; cm.
  Includes bibliographical references.
  ISBN 978-0-8036-4369-7
  I. Title.
  [DNLM: 1. Evidence-Based Practice. 2. Physical Therapy Modalities. 3. Patient Care—methods. 4. Physical Therapist Assistants—standards. WB 460]
  RM700
  615.8'2—dc23
                              2015025818

To Pat for his steadfast love and support; to Drew, Kayla, Shea, and Caitlin for their encouragement; to Ken and Joy for teaching me to always finish what I started; and to Wynn, my newest inspiration.

The seed of an idea for this textbook was planted many years ago while I was a physical therapist assistant (PTA) educator. At the time, our program was using many textbooks written specifically for physical therapists (PTs) because they were the only texts available. This made teaching and learning more difficult because I felt it was important to present material from the PTA perspective and within the PTA role. I often found myself wading through massive textbooks that we had adopted and extracting the portions of the text that were relevant for PTA education. Over the years, a number of my peers addressed this challenge by writing textbooks specifically for the PTA and covering a variety of topics. These texts have been beneficial to PTA education by framing the contents within the PTA role in physical therapy and health care, and I applaud the authors for their commitment to PTA education. However, a gap continued to exist in the area of research methods and evidence based practice.

The PT doctoral-level curriculum typically includes courses in research methods as well as exposure to research through student projects or involvement with faculty research. The PTA associate-level curriculum typically does not include these opportunities for students because of the constraints of compressing the critical elements of patient care for PTAs into a 2-year program. Therefore, entry-level PTAs have likely not been exposed to the basic concepts of research methods and evidence based practice. To become effective participants in the profession and effective members of PT/PTA teams, a basic understanding of research methods and concepts of evidence based practice is needed. This text presents an overview of these topics and provides the reader with learning opportunities to develop skills in the evidence based practice process. It provides a variety of learning activities to facilitate the development of skills in clarifying a clinical question and conducting a search for evidence, as well as strategies for appraising the evidence and incorporating evidence into patient care. The chapters include opportunities for practicing at each step along the way.

This text was primarily written for use within an entry-level PTA curriculum, with an aim of presenting material focused on the role of the PTA within physical therapy practice. The text would also be useful as a reference for PTA clinicians who would like to develop their knowledge and skills about evidence based practice. Clinicians in other health-care fields, such as occupational therapy assistants, might also find the text helpful in introducing concepts that are becoming more important within health care practice.

The three chapters in Part One, Overview of Evidence Based Practice, focus on the development of evidence based practice and its importance to the profession and to health care. The components of the evidence based practice process are presented, and consideration of the unique values and circumstances of each patient is emphasized. The overall goal of Part One is familiarizing the PTA with evidence based practice in preparation for more in-depth discussions in the following sections.

Part Two includes five chapters that present a discussion of research concepts and the different types of research likely to be encountered in a search for best available evidence. An introduction to basic research terminology, including sampling, validity, reliability, and research design, is followed by a series of chapters that discuss experimental, exploratory, and descriptive research, systematic reviews, meta-analyses, and clinical practice guidelines. Numerous examples of physical therapy research articles and case scenarios are presented to reinforce the reader's understanding of this complex topic. The overall goal of Part Two is acquainting the PTA with research methods and common research terminology.

Part Three builds on the first two parts of this text and delves into greater detail about the process of evidence based clinical decision-making. The importance of asking the right clinical question is emphasized as the basis for the literature search. Different sources of evidence are described along with a discussion of hierarchies of evidence and why some types of evidence are better than others. A table of search engines and databases is presented along with a discussion of methods for conducting an efficient and effective search. The reader is provided with tools to understand and appraise a research article. The final chapter discusses the process of integrating evidence with the clinician's knowledge and the patient's values while working within the plan of care developed by the PT. The overall goal of Part Three is to provide the PTA, as a part of the PT/PTA team, with practical tools for using evidence in the clinical decision-making process.

Dianne L. Abels, MSPT
Associate Professor, Academic
    Coordinator of Clinical Education
Allied Health/Physical Therapist
    Assistant Program
Black Hawk College
Moline, Illinois

Diana M. Carman, PT, DPT
Director of Clinical Education
Physical Therapist Assistant Program
Athens Technical College
Athens, Georgia

Leslie Ann Helman, DPT
Faculty
Physical Therapist Assistant Program
Cape Girardeau Career & Technology
    Center
Cape Girardeau, Missouri

Heather MacKrell, PT, PhD
Program Director
Health Sciences
Calhoun Community College
Tanner, Alabama

Becky S. McKnight, PT, MS
Co-Owner
Educational Consulting
Reach Consulting
Powersite, Missouri

Jeremy Oldham, MEd, BS, PTA
Academic Clinical Coordinator
    of Education
Physical Therapist Assistant Program
Allegany College of Maryland
Cumberland, Maryland

Ellen P. O'Keefe, PT, DPT
Program Chair
Physical Therapist Assistant Program
Athens Technical College
Athens, Georgia

Carrie Perkins, PTA, ACCE
Physical Therapist Assistant Program
Mohave Community College
Cottonwood, Arizona

Gary Robinson, MS, PT, PCS
Associate Professor–Allied Health
    Department Chair–PTA Program
    Director
Allied Health
Murray State College
Tishomingo, Oklahoma

Stacey Bell Sloas, PT, MSE
Assistant Professor
Physical Therapy
Arkansas State University
State University, Arkansas

Sharon Lynn Suggett , PTA, BS
Coordinator of Clinical Education
Physical Therapist Assistant Program
Victoria College
Victoria, Texas

Brian J Wilkinson, PT, DPT
Physical Therapist, Instructor
Health Professions
Lane Community College
Eugene, Oregon

Jane E. Worley, PT, MS
Director
Physical Therapist Assistant Program
Lake Superior College
Duluth, Minnesota

Part Three: Finding and Utilizing the Evidence, 127

Barbara Gresham, PT, PhD, GCS is an Associate Professor and Director of the Doctor of Physical Therapy Program at University of Mary Hardin(Baylor. She earned her PhD in Physical Therapy at Texas Woman's University, a Master of Science in Biology/Physiology degree at Baylor University, and a Bachelor of Science in Physical Therapy degree at the University of Texas Southwestern Medical Center in Dallas. She previously served for many years as the Director and ACCE for the Physical Therapist Assistant Program at McLennan Community College. Dr. Gresham has practiced in a variety of settings as a therapist and rehabilitation director and is a board-certified clinical specialist in geriatrics. Her clinical interests include geriatrics, rehabilitation following joint replacements, fall prevention, wellness and health promotion, and developing effective PT/PTA teams. She has been an active member of the American Physical Therapy Association since 1979, serving in a variety of capacities at the local, state, and national levels. Dr. Gresham has been a site reviewer for the Commission on Accreditation in Physical Therapy Education since 1990 and served for 7 years as a commissioner.

Part One provides an introduction to evidence based practice (EBP) and lays the groundwork for skill development in the evidence based clinical decision-making process. Chapter 1 defines EBP and describes the development and importance of EBP. Key terminology is introduced, and basic concepts are defined and discussed. Chapter 2 outlines the components of EBP and the steps involved in searching for and utilizing evidence. Chapter 3 discusses considerations in evidence based clinical decision-making related to the unique values and circumstances of each patient.

The overall goal of Part One is to familiarize the physical therapist assistant (PTA) with EBP in preparation for more in-depth discussions in the following parts. Although the primary purpose is focused on PTAs, some of the conversations in these chapters and throughout the text relate to the physical therapist (PT) and to the PT/PTA team in order to provide a comprehensive discussion of physical therapy practice. Throughout the text, the role of the PTA in evidence based physical therapy practice will be emphasized.

- Chapter 1: The Development of Evidence Based Practice
- Chapter 2: Components of Evidence Based Practice
- Chapter 3: Patient Values and Circumstances in Evidence Based Practice

The Development of Evidence Based Practice

Chapter at a Glance

Learning Outcomes

After reading this chapter, the reader will be able to:

· Define evidence based practice (EBP).
· Describe the development of EBP and the principles on which it is based.
· Define key terminology related to EBP.
· Explain the importance of EBP to health care in general and physical therapy in particular.
· Identify barriers to the utilization of EBP and strategies to address them.
· Identify key documents within the physical therapy profession that address EBP.
· Discuss the role of the physical therapist assistant (PTA) in EBP.

Key Terms

· Applied research
· Basic research
· Clinical practice guidelines
· Clinical research
· Evidence
· Evidence based medicine
· Evidence based practice
· Randomized controlled trial (RCT)
· Systematic review

◘ FOOD FOR THOUGHT

You are working as a PTA in a busy outpatient orthopedic practice. At least once a week you have a conference with each physical therapist (PT) to discuss the patients you are treating. Today you are meeting with Jason, a new graduate PT who has been in practice for just 2 months. Jason evaluated a patient who was referred to therapy following a grade 3 ankle sprain, and then he placed the patient on your schedule for follow-up treatment. The plan of care included ice massage, therapeutic exercise for flexibility and strengthening, and functional activities for progressive weight-bearing. You have treated the patient several times and have noticed that the patient is experiencing a lot of pain and swelling. You are planning to ask Jason if it would be appropriate to add electrical stimulation to the plan of care to address pain and swelling.

Questions to consider:

· Is your rationale for wanting to add electrical stimulation based on current evidence?
· How would you determine whether the evidence supports the use of electrical stimulation for this type of injury?
· Would it be appropriate for you to use electrical stimulation as an intervention with this patient without discussing it with the therapist? Why or why not?

Introduction

Physical therapists (PTs) and physical therapist assistants (PTAs) are part of a dynamic and evolving profession. The PT role has changed over the years from a technician performing treatment directed by a physician to a health-care professional with direct access to patients in many states. The American Physical Therapy Association (APTA) Vision 2020 Statement projected the future role of the PT as the autonomous practitioner of choice for issues related to movement and function. The PTA is an integral part of the PT/PTA team and assists the PT in delivering patient care. The APTA Vision 2020 Statement described the expectation that "physical therapists and physical therapist assistants will render evidence based services throughout the continuum of care."[1] In 2013, the APTA House of Delegates adopted a new Vision Statement for the Physical Therapy Profession.[2] This vision statement continues to emphasize the utilization of evidence in physical therapy practice as well as the generation, validation, and dissemination of evidence. The term *evidence based practice* (EBP) is now widely used in health care, but it may not always be clear exactly what the term means. What information is considered evidence? What other factors, if any, should be considered in EBP? Does utilization of evidence in clinical practice by PTs and PTAs improve patient care?

Evidence based practice has been defined as the integration of the best available research evidence with the clinician's expertise and the patient's individual values and circumstances.[3,4] **Evidence** refers to the available body of scientific research literature, such as journal articles of original research. If you have looked at a copy of the *Physical Therapy Journal* and read a research article, then you have seen an example of evidence. Perhaps the article was somewhat difficult to read, particularly if you have not completed a course in statistics or research methods. It would be quicker to simply read the abstract, which is typically found at the beginning of the article, to decide if the research findings would be helpful to you. However, the abstract cannot paint the whole picture because an abstract is merely a summary of the full article. In order to fully utilize evidence in providing patient care, the clinician must be able to read and appraise a research article. An article typically includes a background review of the literature, a description of the materials and methods used, the results, and the author's discussion of findings and conclusion. This chapter will introduce you to basic terminology related to EBP and will provide an introduction to the development of EBP in physical therapy. All of the concepts and terminology will be explored in greater detail in later chapters.

Development of Evidence Based Practice

The concept of EBP originated in the field of medicine. Evidence based medicine was introduced in the early 1970s as a model for physicians to blend the areas of research and clinical practice in order to improve the quality of patient care. **Evidence based medicine** was defined as "the conscientious, explicit, and judicious use of current best evidence in making decisions about the care of individual patients."[5] Using the model of evidence based medicine, physicians were encouraged to integrate their clinical expertise with the best available evidence to provide quality patient care. Critics of evidence based medicine argued that this model of practice would result in a cookbook approach to medicine. For example, if the evidence supported a particular intervention for a diagnosis, that intervention might be used for every patient with that diagnosis regardless of the physician's skill and knowledge or the patient's specific circumstances. Supporters argued, however, that evidence based medicine required the physician to consider the current best evidence in combination with the physician's clinical experience and the patient's preferences. Instead of a cookbook approach, this would result in an individualized approach to patient care that would in turn result in better patient outcomes.

Learning Task

You have gone to see your primary care physician during the early fall months for a routine examination. Because you are a health-care worker, your physician recommended an influenza vaccination. Access the Internet and go to the Centers for Disease Control and Prevention (CDC) website (www.cdc.gov). Locate the CDC guidelines for influenza vaccinations for adults and answer the following questions:

- What was the basis for the physician's recommendation?
- Is there evidence to support the recommendation?
- Do you think the physician would have made the same recommendation if you worked in a field other than health care?

The evidence based medicine model has become ingrained in the practice of medicine over the past 40 years. During that time, the concepts have spread to other health-care disciplines such as physical therapy, nursing, mental health, and social work. As the concepts of evidence based medicine expanded into other areas of health care, the term *evidence based practice* began to be used. Evidence based practice (EBP) requires the incorporation of best available evidence with a clinician's expertise and the patient's individual values and circumstances (Fig. 1.1). The integration of all three aspects is a key consideration. A clinician relying primarily on evidence might be inclined to apply the same interventions to all patients regardless of patient differences or patient preferences. A clinician relying primarily on clinical experience might be using outdated evaluation or treatment techniques, particularly with the rapid advancements in health care. Portney and Watkins recommended *evidence based decision-making* as a more

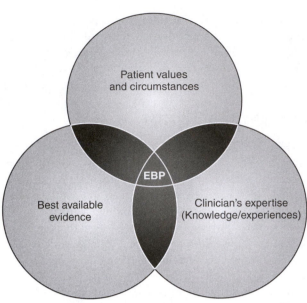

Figure 1.1 Evidence based practice requires the incorporation of best available evidence with a clinician's expertise and the patient's individual values and circumstances.

accurate term because the clinician must consider all relevant information and evidence in making clinical decisions.[6] Two key aspects of promoting EBP in physical therapy are the availability of scientific research related to physical therapy and the ability of clinicians to utilize the evidence in practice.

In order for a profession to embrace the model of EBP, a wide-ranging collection of published scientific research is necessary. Scientific research can be broadly categorized as either basic research or applied research.[6] **Basic research**, sometimes called *bench research*, can be defined as fundamental research that investigates core concepts. The purpose of basic research is to further knowledge and answer basic scientific questions. It typically consists of nonhuman studies and is conducted in a laboratory setting. An example of this type of research would be a laboratory study to investigate the role of a particular enzyme during a muscle contraction in mice. **Applied research** can be defined as research that seeks to solve practical problems, and it is usually grounded in basic science research. Applied research is conducted under actual situational conditions rather than in a laboratory setting. Clinical research is one type of applied research. **Clinical research** consists of studies that directly or indirectly involve humans as subjects and typically investigates diagnosis or treatment of health problems. An example of this type of research would be an intervention study that is investigating the use of backward walking on a treadmill in patients with a diagnosis of stroke.

Medicine has a long history of conducting and disseminating both basic and clinical research. Physical therapy has not historically had the same depth and breadth of research evidence. The first two reported research trials in physical therapy were published in 1929 and 1931, and both investigated electrotherapy.[7] By 1960, only 15 randomized controlled trials directly related to physical therapy had been published. A **randomized controlled trial (RCT)** is defined as a study in which subjects are assigned randomly to groups to receive one of several interventions, with one group serving as a control group. RCTs are considered the gold standard of clinical trials because they compare an experimental intervention with a placebo or standard intervention in a controlled manner.

Over the next 40 years, the number of reported clinical trials dramatically increased as the physical therapy profession moved toward expanding the base of physical therapy knowledge (Fig. 1.2). The body of research in physical therapy now includes a large variety of sources such as RCTs, systematic reviews, and evidence based clinical practice guidelines.[7] A **systematic review** is a specific type of literature review that focuses on a research or clinical question and pulls together all of the available evidence that is applicable to the question. The review will attempt to identify all relevant studies, particularly focusing on RCTs. The authors will assess the quality of the identified studies using a rigid checklist or guideline. The highest quality and most relevant studies will be selected, and a summary of those results will be presented. The systematic review is a key component of EBP because it provides a concise means of reviewing the evidence.

Another key component of EBP is clinical practice guidelines. **Clinical practice guidelines** are recommendations for the diagnosis, treatment, or prevention of healthcare problems that are typically developed by a panel of experts and are based on the best current evidence.[7] These guidelines support clinicians in the clinical decision-making process. Some types of evidence are considered stronger than others in EBP, and Figure 1.3 depicts a hierarchy of evidence. The sources at the bottom of the pyramid are more likely to be biased, whereas the sources at the top of the pyramid are less likely to be biased and therefore are considered the best sources of evidence. Levels of evidence will be discussed in greater detail in Part Two of this text.

Although the body of research has grown, physical therapy clinicians may not be utilizing the information as a basis for clinical decision-making. A 2003 study of PTs investigated the attitudes, knowledge, and beliefs of PTs related to EBP.[8] Most respondents

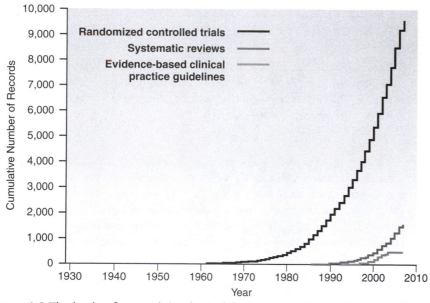

Figure 1.2 The body of research in physical therapy grew slowly during the first decades following the publication of the first two research trials in 1929 and 1931. Since 1980, the profession has seen an exponential increase in the number of RCTs. *Source:* Maher CG, Moseley AM, Sherrington C, Elkins MR, Herbert RD. A description of the trials, reviews, and practice guidelines indexed in the PEDro database. *Phys Ther.* 2008;88(9):1068-1077, with permission from the American Physical Therapy Association. Copyright © 2008 American Physical Therapy Association.

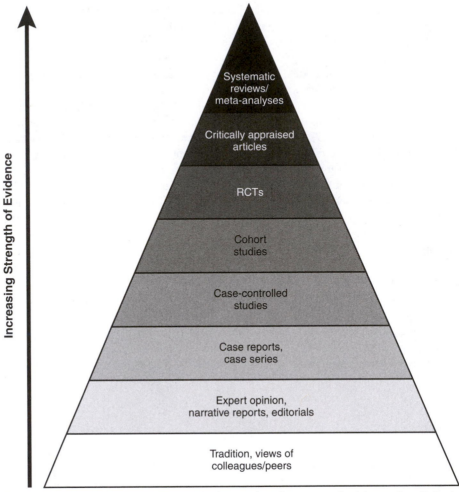

Figure 1.3 The pyramid represents the hierarchy of sources of evidence for clinical decision-making. The higher levels on the pyramid represent stronger levels of evidence. RCTs, randomized controlled trials.

indicated that they had the skills and knowledge necessary to search for and appraise research literature. However, 84% of therapists indicated that they needed to increase the use of evidence in their daily practice, and 74% reported using research literature in the clinical decision-making process five or fewer times per month. PTs with a baccalaureate professional degree were significantly less likely to have training and confidence in their skills than therapists with a postbaccalaureate professional degree. EBP was not widely incorporated into physical therapy education programs in the United States until the past couple of decades. A large number of therapists graduated from entry-level programs before these concepts were commonly taught. Some PTA programs do not include the concepts of EBP in their curriculum or provide only limited content. Therefore a significant number of currently practicing physical therapy clinicians may lack adequate training and skill in EBP.

EBP has sometimes been referred to as a three-legged stool (Fig. 1.4). The three legs of the stool represent the primary components of EBP. One leg represents the body of research available to the clinician, another leg represents the clinician's clinical experience and knowledge, and the third leg represents the patient's values,

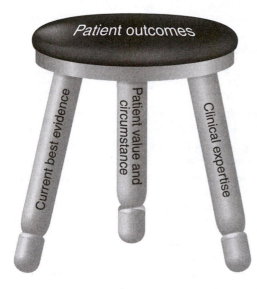

Figure 1.4 Evidence based practice can be represented by a three-legged stool. Each leg represents a component of evidence based practice, with the seat representing patient outcomes.

preferences, beliefs, and circumstances. The three legs together support the seat of the stool, which represents the outcomes of patient care. In any given patient-clinician interaction, the amount of weight supported by each leg may vary. As an example, if a clinician sees a patient with very unusual signs and symptoms, the clinician may find little information in the body of research. In that situation, the clinician must rely more on clinical experience and patient circumstance to determine the best plan of care. For a more common diagnosis, the amount of evidence available will likely be much greater and will provide more support for clinical decision-making.

Why Is Evidence Based Practice Important?

Goals of using evidence in providing health-care services include (1) improving the quality of patient care, (2) standardizing certain aspects of care, and (3) achieving the best possible patient outcomes. The emphasis on EBP in health care during the past couple of decades has resulted from a variety of factors. Increased accountability of health-care providers and health-care institutions has led to a pursuit for clinical practice guidelines and other decision-making guidelines that are based on research. As information about medical errors and variability in the management of patient conditions has become readily available to the public, health-care providers have faced increased pressure to justify the rationale for clinical decisions. As health-care costs continue to rise, physical therapy clinicians may experience difficulties with reimbursement for tests and interventions that are not based on the best available evidence.[9]

In the early years of physical therapy, clinicians were more likely to rely on authority or tradition in making clinical decisions. Some interventions were chosen because they were accepted as the standard, even if they were not based on evidence. In today's health-care environment, however, physical therapy clinicians must be able to articulate evidence based clinical decisions to patients and their families, physicians, other health-care providers, policy makers, and third-party payers.[10] As independent practitioners, PTs must incorporate the best available evidence into the evaluation and development of the patient's plan of care as well as treatment interventions and all other aspects of care. The therapist should be able to clearly explain to the patient the scientific rationale for clinical decisions. Just as important, the PTA should incorporate the most current evidence into treatment interventions and patient management and must be able to provide clear explanations for clinical decisions as well.

A large amount of information is available through media sources today, and patients are more informed. You are likely aware, though, that not all of the information available is accurate. Patients may request a specific type of treatment modality or ask about a specific product because they saw it on television or read about it on the Internet. The PT and PTA must be well informed in order to help patients understand that the information they bring may not be accurate or may not be relevant to their particular circumstance.

Insurance companies and third-party payers continually search for ways to reduce costs, and one way to control costs is to limit reimbursement. As a result, these organizations are taking a closer look at the services for which they are willing to reimburse.[11] Third-party payers have recognized that there is a lot of variation from one area of the country to the next (and even from one physical therapy clinic to the next) in the type of interventions and frequency of physical therapy services provided for a single diagnosis. Variations in patient outcomes and cost of care cannot always be explained by patients' demographic or clinical characteristics. As a result, some insurance companies have begun to deny payment for specific physical agents or treatment interventions because of lack of supporting evidence. This environment requires the use of treatment measures that can be justified by evidence.

Barriers to Evidence Based Practice

As you learn more about EBP, you may think it is reasonable that patient care should be based on current research evidence. Not all health-care providers have fully embraced the concept, and the reasons are varied. One major barrier that has been identified is the time required to review the literature. Most respondents in the previously cited 2003 study identified insufficient time as one of the top three barriers to utilizing evidence based principles (Fig. 1.5).[8] How can a busy clinician find time during a typical work week to read journal articles or search the literature for answers to clinical questions? Therapists and assistants must be educated in methods to locate research literature because using specific strategies can significantly reduce the amount of time required. Clinicians who utilize evidence in day-to-day patient care become much more proficient and efficient in their efforts over time. The use of systematic reviews and clinical practice guidelines can also significantly reduce the time required in locating research evidence. Another barrier is the difficulty in reading and interpreting scientific articles as well as difficulty in appraising the quality of the literature. Education in basic research methodologies and EBP principles is critical to prepare clinicians to routinely utilize evidence in clinical decision-making. Continuing education courses on these topics are available for clinicians who do not feel adequately trained or prepared. Limited access to databases has been cited as a barrier, particularly by therapists working in subacute rehabilitation and skilled nursing facilities. However, access to professional journals and online databases is readily available through membership in professional associations as well as many local and school libraries.

Support for Evidence Based Practice

The APTA plays an important role in the advancement of EBP in physical therapy. The APTA has adopted a number of documents that outline expectations related to EBP. Vision 2020, which was adopted by the APTA House of Delegates in 2000, outlined the expectation that PTs and PTAs will provide evidence based physical therapy services.[1] The newer Vision Statement for the Physical Therapy Profession continues to emphasize

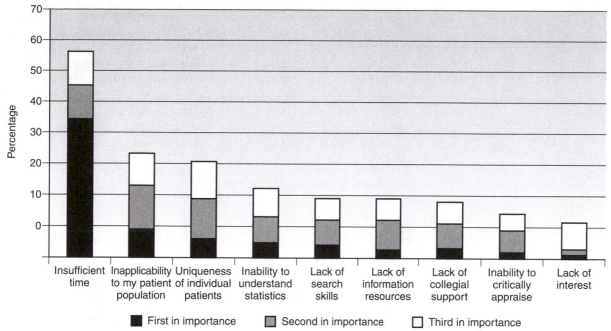

Figure 1.5 Self-reported rankings of barriers to evidence based practice. *Source:* Jette DU, Bacon K, Batty C, et al. Evidence based practice: beliefs, attitudes, knowledge and behaviors of physical therapists. *Phys Ther.* 2003;83;786-805, with permission from the American Physical Therapy Association. Copyright © 2003 American Physical Therapy Association.

best practice and the use of evidence in patient care.[2] The APTA House of Delegates adopted a position statement in 2006 that describes the association's support for the development and utilization of EBP (Box 1.1).[12] The APTA *Guide to Physical Therapist Practice* provides a description of PT practice including preferred practice patterns and the tests, measures, and interventions used.[13] The *Guide* emphasizes the importance of reliable and valid tests and measures and the use of evidence based interventions. The APTA has also developed a number of online tools that provide access to databases, promote the development of clinical practice documents, and educate members about EBP. The APTA includes a number of practice sections, such as the Section on Geriatrics and the Acute Care Section. Many of the practice sections provide online tools for section members that promote EBP. Examples of the APTA and section tools will be described and utilized throughout this text.

The Commission on Accreditation in Physical Therapy Education (CAPTE) is the organization that accredits PT and PTA programs. The commission provides specific criteria that must be met in order for an educational program to become and remain accredited. The *Evaluative Criteria for Physical Therapist Assistant Programs* outlines expectations for the entry-level PTA in relation to utilizing evidence in patient care.[14] The entry-level PTA is expected to be able to read and understand the literature. In addition, the entry-level PTA is expected to be able to identify and integrate appropriate evidence based resources in the clinical decision-making process within the plan of care developed by the PT. Other criteria, although not explicitly referring to evidence based decision-making, would require the PTA to maintain current knowledge of the evidence. For example, one criterion states that the entry-level PTA is expected to adjust interventions within the plan of care in response to patient clinical indications. In order

> **Box 1.1** | **American Physical Therapy Association Position Statement on Evidence Based Practice**
>
> **Evidence Based Practice HOD P06-06-12-08 [Position] [Initial HOD P06-99-17-21]**
> To promote improved quality of care and patient/client outcomes, the American Physical Therapy Association supports and promotes the development and utilization of evidence based practice that includes the integration of best available research, clinical expertise, and patient values and circumstances related to patient/client management, practice management, and health policy decision making.
>
> *Source:* American Physical Therapy Association (www.apta.org).

to appropriately adjust interventions, the PTA must have an understanding of the most current best evidence.

Role of the PTA in Evidence Based Practice

Much of the conversation about EBP deals with diagnosis and prognosis, test and measures for examination/evaluation, and selection of interventions in the development of a plan of care. These components of physical therapy practice are the responsibility of the PT. How does the PTA fit into the EBP picture? Figure 1.6 illustrates the role of the PTA within physical therapy patient management, although there may be some variability based on state jurisdictions and regulatory guidelines. Physical therapy patient management consists of six elements: Examination (which includes Tests and Measures), Evaluation, Diagnosis, Prognosis, Intervention, and Outcome. The role of the PTA falls primarily within the Intervention element. For purposes of illustration, the component of Tests and Measures has been separated from the Examination element. PTAs are expected to be able to competently perform selected data collection skills, which are encompassed under Tests and Measures, within the context of carrying out interventions and ensuring that patient goals are met. PTAs do not, however, conduct other elements of Examination. PTAs share responsibility for Outcome by ensuring that patient goals established in the plan of care by the PT are being met. The level of involvement within each element depends on a number of factors, including the patient care setting, the level of complexity of the patient, the experience and skill level of the PTA, and the experience of the PT.

The PTA should assume responsibility for staying current with research literature that addresses interventions. Although the PTA will not be selecting the interventions for the patient's plan of care, the PTA must be able to clearly communicate with the PT and the patient about the purpose of the intervention, risks and benefits, and evidence supporting its use. At times, the PTA might recommend a different intervention to the therapist if the patient is not responding as expected to an intervention in the plan of care. The PTA must also be knowledgeable about specific data collection tests and measures, including reliability and validity. CAPTE criteria include an expectation that entry-level PTAs will perform selected components of data collection necessary for carrying out the plan of care.[14] PTAs may also be called on by the PT to assist with data collection during an examination. In addition, PTAs should be knowledgeable about outcome measures that can help determine how well a patient is progressing toward the goals established by the PT. All of these responsibilities include an expectation that the PTA will incorporate the best available evidence in providing patient care.

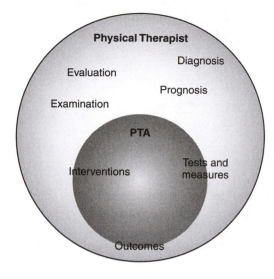

Figure 1.6 A representation of physical therapy patient management reflecting the responsibilities of the physical therapist (PT) and the role of the physical therapist assistant (PTA). The PT is responsible for all aspects of patient management. The PTA assists the PT with interventions, tests and measures, and shares responsibility for ensuring that the expected patient outcomes are met.

SUMMARY

EBP is the integration of the best available evidence with the clinician's expertise and the patient's values and circumstances. PTs and PTAs are expected to provide evidence based services to patients. A broad base of published scientific research is necessary to support EBP, and clinicians must be educated in strategies for reading, interpreting, and appraising scientific literature. Goals of EBP include improving the quality of patient care, standardizing care, and achieving the best possible patient outcomes. Barriers to EBP have been identified and include limited time to review the literature, difficulty in reading and interpreting articles, and limited access to databases. Strategies to overcome these barriers include educating clinicians in search strategies, continuing education in interpreting and appraising scientific literature, and promoting membership in professional organizations that provide database access. PTAs play an important role in EBP as part of the PT/PTA team and should assume responsibility for staying current with research literature.

● Case Scenario

You are a PTA working in a community hospital that has a total joint program. Six months ago the Total Joint Program Committee, with input from the orthopedic surgeons, decided to stop using continuous passive motion (CPM) units following total knee arthroplasty. Some surgeons will use a positioning pillow that holds the knee in extension and keeps the leg elevated following surgery, while other surgeons have chosen to use no device.

One of the PTs evaluated a patient this morning on postoperative day 1 following total knee arthroplasty. The therapist asked you to treat the patient after lunch for exercise and gait training activities. When you arrive in the patient's room, the patient asks you why she has to keep her leg positioned on the pillow. She states that she had her other knee replaced last year and they used a CPM. She is concerned that the pillow "doesn't do anything." How would you respond?

CASE QUESTIONS

1. Would you be able to explain the rationale for using this type of positioning pillow rather than a CPM?

_____

_____

2. Is there evidence that supports discontinuing use of the CPM?

_____

_____

3. Is there evidence that supports the use of the positioning pillow?

_____

_____

Learning Task
Using Google Scholar (http://scholar.google.com), find a research article that addresses the use of CPM or extension positioning pillow following total knee arthroplasty. Read your article and be prepared to participate in group discussion with classmates. Note the source of your article and see if you can categorize your article based on the hierarchy of evidence in Figure 1.1.

Review Activities

1. In your own words, define evidence based practice.

   _____

   _____

   _____

   _____

2. List three goals of evidence based practice.

   _____

   _____

   _____

   _____

3. List three barriers to evidence based practice and a strategy for each barrier.

   _____

   _____

   _____

   _____

4. Briefly explain the concept of the three-legged stool in evidence based practice.

   _____

   _____

   _____

   _____

5. List three professional documents or statements that support evidence based physical therapy.

   _____

   _____

   _____

   _____

6. Identify the elements of physical therapy patient management in which the PTA is involved.

_____

_____

_____

_____

MATCHING

_____ 1. Evidence

_____ 2. Basic research

_____ 3. Applied research

_____ 4. Clinical research

_____ 5. RCTs

_____ 6. Systematic reviews

_____ 7. Clinical practice guideline

A. Literature review with synthesis of results

B. Research involving human subjects

C. Body of scientific research literature

D. Evidence based recommendation from experts

E. Aimed at increasing scientific knowledge without attempting to solve problems

F. Type of study with randomly assigned subjects, considered gold standard of clinical research

G. Research conducted under actual conditions

■ References

1. American Physical Therapy Association. Vision 2020. www.apta.org/Vision2020. Accessed June 24, 2015.
2. American Physical Therapy Association. Vision statement. www.apta.org/Vision. Accessed June 24, 2015.
3. Fetters L, Tilson J. *Evidence Based Physical Therapy*. Philadelphia, PA: FA Davis; 2012.
4. Kronenfeld M, Stephenson PL, Nail-Chiwetalu B, et al. Review for librarians of evidence-based practice in nursing and the allied health professions in the United States. *J Med Libr Assoc*. 2007;95(4):394-407.
5. Sackett DL, Rosenberg WM, Gray JA, Haynes RB, Richardson WS. Evidence based medicine: what it is and what it isn't. *Br Med J (Clin Res Ed)*. 1996;312(7023):71-72.
6. Portney LG, Watkins MP. *Foundations of Clinical Research: Applications to Practice*. Upper Saddle River, NJ: Pearson Education; 2008.
7. Maher CG, Moseley AM, Sherrington C, Elkins MR, Herbert RD. A description of the trials, reviews, and practice guidelines indexed in the PEDro database. *Phys Ther*. 2008;88(9):1068-1077.
8. Jette DU, Bacon K, Batty C, et al. Evidence-based practice: beliefs, attitudes, knowledge and behaviors of physical therapists. *Phys Ther*. 2003;83:786-805.
9. Jewell DV. *Guide to Evidence-Based Physical Therapist Practice*. 3rd ed. Burlington, MA: Jones & Bartlett Learning; 2015.

10. Tugwell PS, Santesso NA, O'Connor AM, Wilson AJ. Knowledge translation for effective consumers. *Phys Ther*. 2007;87(12):1728.
11. Chan F, Rosenthal DA, Pruett SR. Evidence-based practice in the provision of rehabilitation services. *J Rehabil*. 2008;74(2):3.
12. American Physical Therapy Association. Policy on evidence based practice. http://www.apta.org/uploadedFiles/APTAorg/About_Us/Policies/Practice/ EvidenceBasedPractice.pdf#search=%22evidence based practice policy%22. Accessed December 3, 2012.
13. American Physical Therapy Association. *Guide to Physical Therapist Practice*. 2nd ed. Alexandria, VA: APTA; 2003.
14. Commission on Accreditation in Physical Therapy Education (CAPTE). *Evaluative Criteria—PTA Programs*. Alexandria, VA: CAPTE; 2013.

Components of Evidence Based Practice

Learning Outcomes

After reading this chapter, the reader will be able to:

· Define the three key components of evidence based practice (EBP).
· Describe the five steps of the EBP process.
· Identify the meaning of the acronym PICO.
· Select key search terms from a clinical question.
· Explain the rationale for critically appraising evidence.
· Discuss specific considerations for determining the relevance and quality of evidence.

Key Terms

· Abstract
· Clinical question
· Clinician
· Database
· Meta-analysis
· Peer-reviewed research
· PICO
· Research hypothesis
· Research question
· Search engine
· Shared decision-making

■ FOOD FOR THOUGHT

You are a physical therapist assistant working in home health care, and you have been treating a 78-year-old woman twice a week for the past 3 weeks. Her primary diagnosis is general debility with a history of multiple recent falls, and she has a fear of falling again because she lives alone. The patient's plan of care includes progressive resistance exercise, gait training, and balance activities with goals of improving the patient's strength, balance, and endurance. The patient's strength and endurance are improving, but her balance is not progressing as expected. The plan of care does not include specific balance activities, so you decide that you need to adjust the balance exercises on your next visit.

Questions to consider:

· What would be your best option for locating current best evidence on balance interventions?

· Would it be important to discuss any changes you make with the supervising therapist? Why or why not?

· Would it be important to explain your rationale for any changes to the patient? Why or why not?

Introduction

Sackett defined evidence based practice (EBP) as "the integration of the best available research evidence with the clinician's expertise and the patient's individual values and circumstances."[1] The three components based upon this definition include (1) the research evidence, (2) the clinician's expertise, and (3) the patient's values and circumstances (Fig. 2.1). (The term **clinician** can be broadly defined as an individual who has

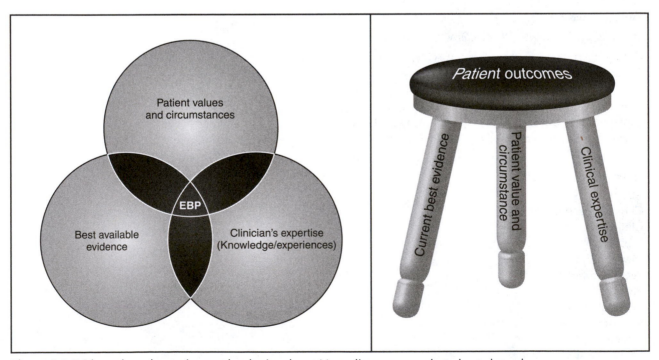

Figure 2.1 Evidence based practice can be depicted as a Venn diagram or a three-legged stool.

patient care responsibilities. In this text, we will use the term *clinician* to refer to the physical therapist or the physical therapist assistant.) You will recall from Chapter 1 that the three components of EBP were illustrated by a Venn diagram and as a three-legged stool. Which component is the most important? Because physical therapy is a profession that emphasizes patient-centered care, one could argue that the patient component is the most important component. Others might argue that the best available evidence or the skill and knowledge of the clinician would be the most important. Still others might argue that all three components are equally important in achieving the best outcomes. The primary consideration, perhaps, is that all three components are critical and must be integrated in order to achieve the best outcome for each patient.

Patient Values and Circumstances

Every patient with whom we interact brings a unique set of values, beliefs, circumstances, and preferences (Fig. 2.2).[2] Although two patients of the same age may have an identical diagnosis, each is likely to approach the diagnosis from a different perspective. Think about the patient who believes there is a pill or medical treatment that can fix any problem compared with the patient who has a distrust of medications and health care in general and believes in home remedies or faith healing. A patient with a recent spinal cord injury may refuse to consider purchasing a wheelchair and other equipment because of a strong belief that he will be able to walk again very soon. Based on a patient's culture, a female patient may not be open to considering aquatic therapy because of her concern for exposing too much of her body, particularly with a male clinician. A patient may not have the financial resources available to purchase a piece of equipment that has been recommended for use at home. All of the unique aspects of the patient, including patient choice, must be considered in EBP.

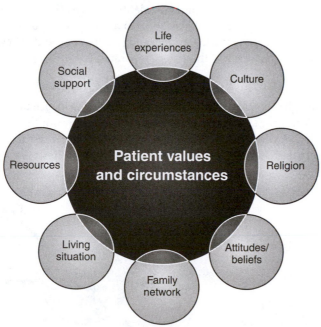

Figure 2.2 A variety of life experiences, situations, and conditions contribute to the patient's perspective as part of evidence based practice.

Clinician Expertise

The base of a clinician's knowledge is shaped during the formal training process in preparation for practice (Fig. 2.3). This would include the educational program that combines classroom learning opportunities with clinical learning opportunities. The key measurement of a clinician's entry-level knowledge is the licensing examination that must be passed in order to enter practice. However, this is only the beginning of the clinician's knowledge and experience. The practice setting chosen by the clinician can in many ways define the breadth and depth of a clinician's experience. A therapist or assistant who chooses an outpatient spine clinic has the potential to gain a deep body of knowledge and experience related to spine conditions and diagnoses. One who chooses a trauma center has the potential to develop a broad body of knowledge and experience because of exposure to a wide variety of patients and diagnoses. The clinician determines the quality of the knowledge gained by making the most of the opportunities provided. If clinicians are doing the same thing with each patient over and over, and not challenging themselves to grow and learn, they are not benefiting from the experiences being presented.

Research Evidence

The body of research evidence that is available to the clinician continues to grow as the emphasis on EBP in physical therapy increases. The body of research available at this time can seem overwhelming to many clinicians (Fig. 2.4). It can be a time-consuming task to read through journal articles or other sources to find the information you are looking for. How do you know exactly what to look for? To find the best information, a clinician should follow the EBP process.

Steps in the Evidence Based Practice Process

The process of EBP includes five commonly identified steps (Fig. 2.5).[3,4] These steps are (1) formulating a focused clinical question, (2) locating the evidence, (3) critically appraising the evidence, (4) applying evidence to patient care, and (5) evaluating the process.[2] We will examine each of these steps separately.

Step 1: Formulate a Focused Clinical Question

Developing the right clinical question is critical to finding evidence that will be useful in the clinical decision-making process. A clinical question is not the same thing as a research question. A **research question** provides the basis for a research study and is sometimes restated as a research hypothesis. A **research hypothesis** is a statement that

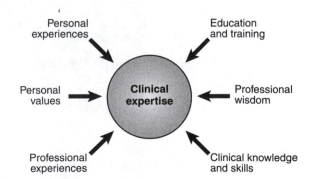

Figure 2.3 A variety of professional and life experiences contribute to the clinician's expertise.

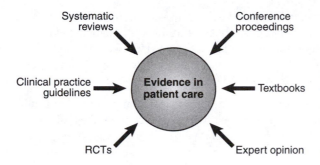

Figure 2.4 Examples of some of the diverse sources of evidence that contribute to evidence based practice. RCTs, randomized controlled trials.

proposes or predicts the relationship between variables before a study being conducted. Both the research question and research hypothesis identify variables to be studied. For example, if you were interested in studying the effect of aerobic exercise on cognition in patients with Parkinson disease, you might ask the question, "Does aerobic exercise improve cognition in patients with Parkinson disease?" or "Does forced aerobic exercise improve cognition more than self-paced aerobic exercise in patients with Parkinson disease?" These questions could also be written as a research hypothesis, such as, "Cognitive function will be significantly higher immediately following forced aerobic exercise and at 1 month follow-up compared with self-paced aerobic exercise in patients with Parkinson disease."[5] A research question or hypothesis must be developed in such a way that an answer can be determined using the scientific method. Research questions are not the focus of this text.

A **clinical question**, on the other hand, provides the basis for a literature search to find information relevant to a particular patient situation. Consider the following situation: You are treating a 56-year-old patient with diabetes mellitus who has a foot ulcer that is healing very slowly. You heard one of the therapists talking about a course

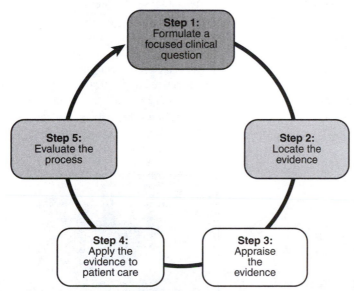

Figure 2.5 The Evidence Based Practice Process includes five steps that facilitate the clinician's ability to answer a clinical question.

she attended that discussed using ultrasound as an intervention in wound care. You want to determine whether ultrasound might be beneficial for your patient before discussing this with the therapist overseeing the patient's care. How would you go about finding the information you need? One commonly used method of developing a good clinical question is to utilize the acronym **PICO** (Fig. 2.6).[6]

- **P – Patient:** Using your patient's diagnosis, describe a group of patients that would include your patient. *Example:* patients with diabetic ulcer(s) of the foot.
- **I – Intervention:** Describe the intervention that you are considering using. *Example:* adding ultrasound to the standard wound care protocol.
- **C – Comparison Intervention** (or **Control**): Describe the main alternative to the intervention you are considering. *Example:* standard wound care protocol alone.
- **O – Outcome**: Describe what would be accomplished, or the outcome that you would like to see for your patient. *Example:* faster wound healing.

After you have addressed each of these four areas, you can put them together to develop your clinical question: "For patients with diabetic ulcer of the foot, would adding ultrasound to the standard wound care protocol compared with using standard wound care protocol alone result in faster wound healing?" A focused clinical question is likely to make the rest of the process easier. Chapter 9 will provide more details about developing focused clinical questions.

Step 2: Locate the Evidence

The second step in the process is to conduct a search of the literature. A literature search can be conducted using a variety of search engines and databases. A **search engine** is an information retrieval system that searches electronic databases and other Internet resources.[7] Search engines may require a subscription or membership in a professional association, such as ArticleSearch available through the American Physical Therapy Association, or may be available to anyone, such as Google Scholar or PubMed. A **database** is an organized system containing lists of reference citations and may include the reference summary, the reference summary and abstract, or the full text of the article.[7] An example of a database is the Cochrane Database of Systematic Reviews, which contains a compilation of systematic reviews on a variety of topics. Another example is Medline, which is the database of the National Library of Medicine and provides citations and abstracts for biomedical literature. The Physiotherapy Evidence Database, called PEDro, contains abstracts of randomized controlled trials (RCTs), systematic reviews, and practice guidelines specifically related to physical therapy. Many databases require a subscription by an individual or an organization. Students will typically have access to some of the search engines and databases through the college library system.

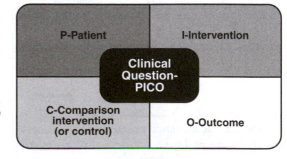

Figure 2.6 The acronym PICO can be used to develop a focused clinical question.

Chapter 11 provides more detail about commonly used search engines and databases for physical therapy and strategies for using them.

To search for literature related to a clinical question, key words or phrases are entered into the search tool. Using the information from a PICO question, it is fairly easy to identify key terms that can be entered. Let's go back to our question: "For patients with *diabetic ulcer* of the foot, would adding *ultrasound* to the standard wound care protocol compared with using standard wound care protocol alone result in faster *wound healing*?" Using PubMed, you could enter the terms *diabetic ulcer, ultrasound,* and *wound healing* for the initial search (Fig. 2.7). You may need to revise your search terms and repeat the search if you are not satisfied with the results of the first search. Figure 2.8 shows the results of the search using PubMed and the search terms *diabetic ulcer, ultrasound,* and *wound healing.*

To most efficiently search for evidence, a clinician should consider including meta-analyses and systematic reviews in the search.[6] As defined in the previous chapter, a *systematic review* is a literature review and summary of existing research evidence that focuses on a specific research or clinical question. A **meta-analysis** is a type of systematic review that pools the data from separate but similar experiments of different researchers and conducts a statistical analysis of the pooled data. Both the systematic review and the meta-analysis are keys to EBP because they provide an effective and efficient method of reviewing a large amount of evidence. If a researcher has recently conducted a systematic review for a question similar to yours, your time may not be well spent by repeating a literature search of the same information.

Another consideration in conducting a literature search is whether to apply any limits to the search. Most search engines allow you to limit your search to a certain time frame, for example, the past 5 or 10 years. You may choose to limit your search to peer-reviewed articles only. **Peer-reviewed research** has been submitted for scrutiny by other

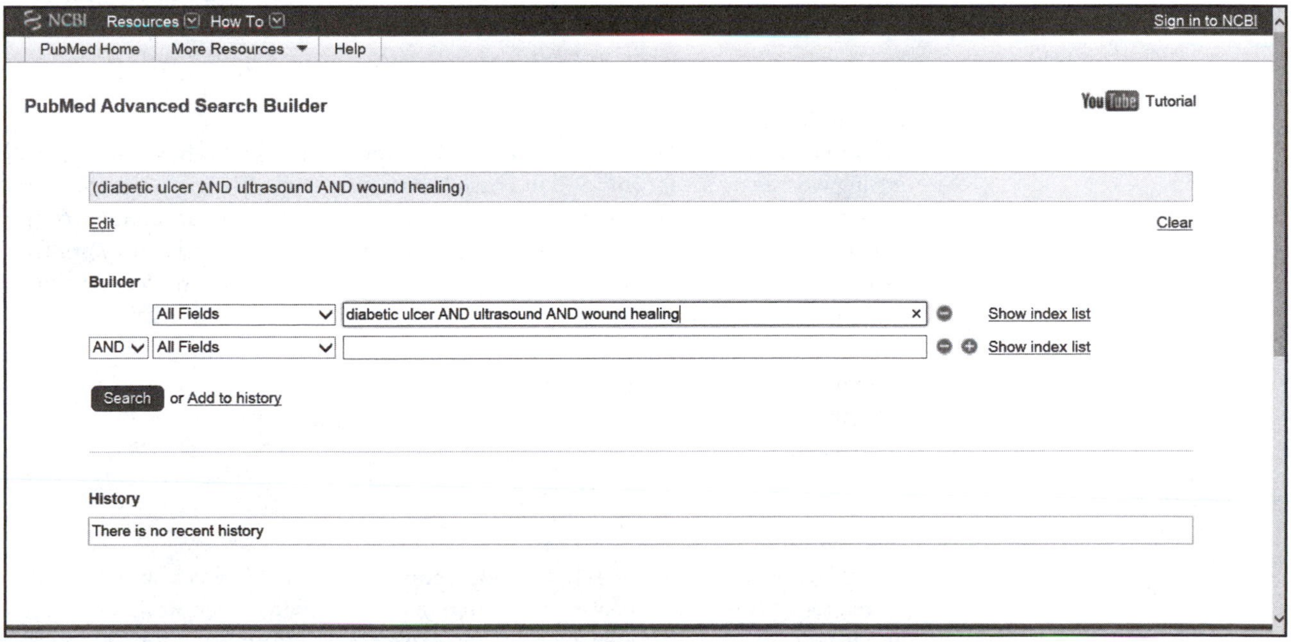

Figure 2.7 PubMed Search Page with search terms entered. *Source:* Screenshot from PubMed (www.pubmed.gov), the U.S. National Library of Medicine, Bethesda, MD, and the National Institute of Health. Accessed January 19, 2015.

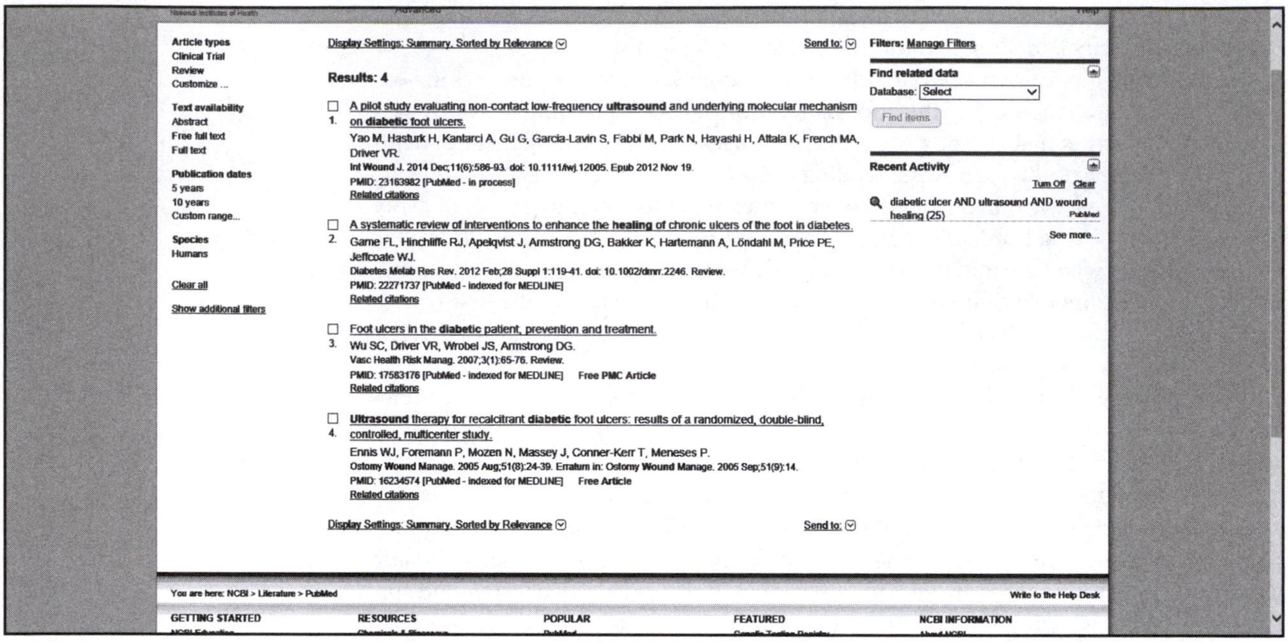

Figure 2.8 PubMed search results. *Source:* Screenshot from PubMed (www.pubmed.gov), the U.S. National Library of Medicine, Bethesda, MD, and the National Institutes of Health. Accessed January 19, 2015.

experts in the field. These experts provide feedback, typically anonymous, on any or all aspects of the research, such as the methods used or the conclusions drawn from the results. This process of critical review before publication is considered the gold standard. Studies that are reported in non–peer-reviewed journals are not necessarily inferior, but they haven't been subjected to the same level of scrutiny.

Learning Task

You are treating a 43-year-old patient with multiple sclerosis who has been experiencing worsening symptoms and increased spasticity. The patient reports that her physician is going to initiate treatment to reduce spasticity using botulinum toxin. You are not familiar with this medical treatment in multiple sclerosis and want to be able to explain to the patient how it might affect her mobility and function in relation to her physical therapy goals. Answer the following questions:

• What is your clinical question?
• What search terms would you use?
• What type of evidence would you search for—RCTs, systematic reviews, meta-analyses?

Learning Task

Using Google Scholar (www.scholar.google.com) or PubMed (www.pubmed.com), search for a research article using the search terms identified earlier. Review the article that you located. Does the article provide enough information for you to be able to explain to your patient how the medical treatment might affect physical therapy treatment and outcome?

Step 3: Critically Appraise the Evidence

After you have completed the literature search, the next step is appraising the search results. This step actually consists of answering two separate questions:

1. Is the study relevant to my clinical question?
2. Is the quality of the study high enough to be helpful?

To save time, the first question listed should be answered first. Trying to determine the quality of a study before you decide if the study is relevant to your question is not an efficient use of time. How do you determine whether research studies or reviews are relevant to your clinical question? Specific factors need to be considered. A research study should include subjects that are similar to your patient in age, diagnosis, and clinical condition (i.e., diabetic ulcer of the foot). A systematic review or meta-analysis should address the specific diagnosis and condition included in your clinical question. The environment can also be an important factor. In other words, a study that investigated individuals in a long-term care facility might not be relevant to your patient who is independent within the community.

Clinicians should not assume that the first article on the list of citations will meet their needs. Instead, they should review a number of the citations that were identified during the search and select results that appear to be most relevant to the specific clinical question. Refer back to Figure 2.8 and review the citations listed. Based on the information provided, can you tell if any of these articles would be relevant to your clinical question? All of the articles seem to be related to the clinical question. The articles cited all address diabetic foot ulcers and include a pilot study, a systematic review, an RCT, and an additional article. To better determine the relevance, it would be helpful to have more information than an article title, such as an abstract. An **abstract** is a summary of a research study, often limited to 250 words or less. It will usually contain the purpose of the study, a brief description of methods and results, and a conclusion. A review of the abstract should provide information about the subjects, which would allow you to determine whether the subjects in the study are similar to your patient in age and diagnosis.

After you have determined that a study or review is relevant to your clinical question, the next step is to appraise the quality of the evidence. To begin appraising the evidence, it might be helpful to determine where the research article falls in the hierarchy of evidence (Fig. 2.9). According to Portney and Watkins, levels of evidence can range from the lowest level of expert opinion to the highest level of a systematic review of RCTs.[7] The clinician should try to find evidence that is located toward the top of the hierarchy of evidence (top of the pyramid), such as systematic reviews and meta-analyses. The clinician must be able to distinguish between different types of articles. For example, the clinician should be able to determine whether an article is a research report, which provides details about a research study or review, or a narrative report, which is a subjective summary of evidence provided from an author's perspective. It may also be helpful to determine whether the evidence was published in a well-respected peer-reviewed journal, which indicates that an article was reviewed by individuals knowledgeable about the topic. The peer-reviewed process doesn't ensure that an article is high quality because some journals may have a less rigorous peer-review process than others. However, journals associated with professional associations tend to be more rigorous. The clinician should also note the authors' affiliations and the source of funding, if any, for the study. Studies that are funded by companies or organizations with a vested interest in the outcome have the potential to be more biased. Parts Two and Three of this text will provide the reader with a discussion of different types of research and methods for understanding a research article, which will prepare the reader to appraise an article with confidence.

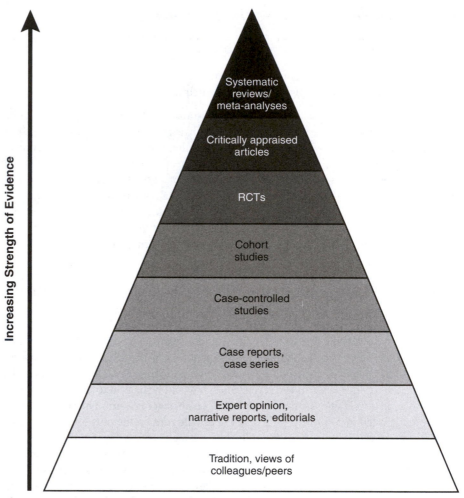

Increasing Strength of Evidence

Systematic reviews/ meta-analyses

Critically appraised articles

RCTs

Cohort studies

Case-controlled studies

Case reports, case series

Expert opinion, narrative reports, editorials

Tradition, views of colleagues/peers

Figure 2.9 Hierarchy of sources of evidence for evidence based practice. RCTs, randomized controlled trials.

Learning Task

Using PubMed (www.pubmed.com), locate one of the articles cited in Figure 2.8. Read the abstract and try to determine whether the abstract provides enough information for you to answer your clinical question. Can you locate the full text of the article? Is the journal peer reviewed? Categorize your article based on the hierarchy of evidence pyramid.

Step 4: Apply the Evidence to Patient Care

The next step in the EBP process is to combine the relevant evidence with the clinician's clinical experience and the patient's specific circumstances. Adams and Drake described shared decision-making as a key component of EBP.[8] **Shared decision-making** was defined as an interactive process of collaboration between the health-care provider and the patient to make health-care decisions. Although the clinician may provide information about the therapy diagnosis, treatment options, and expected outcomes, the patient should provide information about treatment preference and treatment goals.

As an example, the clinician may present the evidence based recommendation of aquatic therapy as the best intervention for a patient's specific type of arthritis. The patient may refuse because of a lifelong fear of water, which requires the clinician to provide alternative interventions. A therapist may present a patient with a plan of care that includes weight loss as one of the goals of treatment in order to control joint pain symptoms. The patient, based on a long struggle with weight control, may reject that goal and focus on other interventions for pain management. Shared decision-making can range from patients desiring to make all of the decisions about their care to patients who want the clinician to make all of the decisions. The most effective decision-making is likely somewhere in the middle of the spectrum, where the clinician and the patient each assume responsibility for their roles in the patient's care. The next chapter discusses patient values and circumstances and their effect on patient care in greater detail.

Step 5: Evaluate the Process

Let's review the EBP process to this point. First, develop a very specific clinical question (PICO) based on a particular patient situation. Next, conduct a literature search to find evidence that will help answer the clinical question. After locating several articles, determine whether the articles are relevant and of sufficient quality to be useful. Then, use the evidence you selected to make a clinical decision in response to the clinical question, taking into account the patient's values and circumstances. The final step is to evaluate the process.[4] It can be helpful to ask yourself questions such as the following:

- *Was the process helpful in answering the clinical question?* Your goal when asking your clinical question was to determine whether ultrasound might be beneficial for your patient before discussing this with the therapist. In this case, you were not relying on your clinical expertise alone to make a decision based on the evidence. If the evidence convinced you that ultrasound would be beneficial for your patient, you would need to discuss this information with the therapist overseeing the patient's care because the therapist is the only provider who can change the plan of care.
- *If the process was not helpful, what might you have done differently?* Asking this question is essential to improving your skills in EBP. The decisions that are made throughout the process can make a difference in the literature search and the usefulness of the studies found. For example, this search only included the PubMed database. If the search had included a database that was physical therapy specific, would different articles have been located? Would the different articles have been more relevant to physical therapy practice?
- *If the process was helpful, what might you do in the future to make the process more efficient or effective?* As you become more involved in EBP, you should become more proficient at performing each step. By answering this question, you can begin to determine which actions you took that were time wasters and which methods of searching were more efficient. For example, you may find that you are most comfortable using one particular search engine. You will also develop greater skill at asking the right clinical question and choosing the best search terms. As you gain experience, you will become more comfortable reading the literature and making a determination about the usefulness and the quality of literature.
- *What was the patient's outcome?* Determining the answer to this question will allow you to expand your clinical knowledge base, regardless of the outcome. The EBP process is exactly that—a process that leads to an outcome. By repeatedly following the EBP process and understanding how the process may have affected the outcome, you are on your way to becoming a more knowledgeable and skilled clinician.

SUMMARY

EBP integrates "the best available research evidence with the clinician's expertise and the patient's individual values and circumstances."[1] The EBP process includes five steps:

- Identify a focused clinical question
- Conduct a literature search
- Critically appraise the literature
- Apply the evidence to individual patients
- Evaluate the EBP process

A common method of developing a good clinical question is to utilize the acronym PICO:

- Patient
- Intervention
- Comparison Intervention (or Control)
- Outcome

A literature search can be conducted using a variety of search engines and databases. After studies have been located, the clinician must critically appraise the literature to determine whether a study is relevant to the clinical question and of sufficient quality to be helpful. The next step is combining the relevant evidence with the clinician's experience and the patient's specific circumstances. Finally, the clinician must evaluate the EBP process by determining whether the process was helpful in answering the clinical question. This will allow the clinician to decide how to make the process more efficient and effective in the future.

● Case Scenario

You are a physical therapist assistant working in an inpatient rehabilitation facility that specializes in the treatment of patients with neurological injuries. You are a member of the facility's Safety and Fall Prevention Committee, which tracks falls and develops and implements fall prevention strategies. Facility policy does not allow the use of restraints except in extreme circumstances. Discussion during the meeting today addressed the increasing fall rate during the past 3 months. One of the committee members pointed out that the staff is often confused about which patients are at greater risk for falling because nursing and therapy use two different fall scales that sometimes provide conflicting results. Nursing has been using the Morse Fall Scale, whereas therapy has been using the Hendrich II Fall Scale. Another concern raised was the lack of uniform fall prevention measures for patients who are at the greatest risk for falling. You have volunteered to conduct a literature search to find evidence related to fall scales, and the committee will then determine which fall scale to adopt.

CASE QUESTIONS

1. What process would you use to develop a clinical question as the basis for the literature search? Write your question now.

_____

_____

2. What search terms would you use for your literature search?

_____

_____

3. Can you find evidence that supports the use of either of the fall scales?

_____

_____

Learning Task

Using PubMed (www.pubmed.com), find a research article that addresses either the Morse Fall Scale or the Hendrich II Fall Scale. Read your article and be prepared to participate in group discussion with classmates to address the case scenario.

Review Activities

1. Identify the three components of evidence based practice.

_____

_____

_____

_____

2. List the five steps of the evidence based practice process.

_____

_____

_____

_____

3. Explain the meaning of the acronym PICO.

_____

_____

_____

_____

4. Identify three factors for determining whether evidence is relevant.

_____

_____

_____

_____

5. List three factors for determining the quality of evidence.

_____

_____

_____

_____

MATCHING

_____ 1. Research question   A. Summary of research article

_____ 2. Research hypothesis   B. Question that can be answered
using scientific method

_____ 3. Clinical question   C. Question to find information about a
patient situation

_____ 4. Search engine   D. System containing citations

_____ 5. Database   E. Statement predicting relationship
                                 of variables in a study

_____ 6. Abstract   F. Information retrieval system

References

1. Sackett DL. Evidence-based medicine. *Semin Perinatol.* 1997:21(1);3-5.
2. Hack LM, Gwyer J. *Evidence Into Practice: Integrating Judgment, Values and Research.* Philadelphia, PA: FA Davis; 2013.
3. Sackett DL, Rosenberg WM, Gray JA, Haynes RB, Richardson WS. Evidence based medicine: what it is and what it isn't. *Br Med J (Clin Res Ed).* 1996;312(7023):71-72.
4. Fetters L, Tilson J. *Evidence Based Physical Therapy.* Philadelphia, PA: FA Davis; 2012.
5. Swank C. *Effect of Aerobic Exercise on Cognition and Sedentary Behavior in Persons With Parkinson Disease.* ProQuest Dissertations and Theses; Dissertations & Theses @ Texas Woman's University, 2011:pg n/a.
6. University of Oxford. Centre for Evidence Based Medicine. http://www.cebm.net/. Accessed January 15, 2013.
7. Portney LG, Watkins MP. *Foundations of Clinical Research: Applications to Practice.* Upper Saddle River, NJ: Pearson Education; 2008.
8. Adams JR, Drake RE. Shared decision making and evidence-based practice. *Community Ment Health J.* 2006:42(1);87-105.

Chapter 3

Patient Values and Circumstances in Evidence Based Practice

Chapter at a Glance

Learning Outcomes

After reading this chapter, the reader will be able to:

· Provide examples of patient values and circumstances that should be considered in evidence based practice.
· Discuss the concept of health literacy and why it is important.
· Identify the key components of patient-centered care and shared decision-making.
· Outline the legal and ethical obligations of clinicians in providing patient care.
· Explain the concept of informed consent.
· Discuss the importance of considering a patient's values and circumstances in clinical decision-making.

Key Terms

· Health literacy
· Informed consent
· Patient-centered care
· Patient circumstances
· Patient values
· Plain language

◘ FOOD FOR THOUGHT

You are a physical therapist assistant working in an orthopedic outpatient clinic, and you recently began treating a 66-year-old patient with a diagnosis of hip fracture with open reduction and internal fixation. His surgery was performed 10 days ago, and he was discharged from the hospital on postoperative day 2. The surgeon recommended home health care, but the patient refused because it would make him feel "helpless." His wife has been driving him to his appointments, and she has expressed concern that he is pushing himself too hard. You have established a good rapport with the patient, who loves to tell jokes and humorous stories. On his fourth clinic visit, you notice that he is much quieter than usual and appears to be having difficulty completing his exercises. When you question him about his pain level, he reports that he quit taking his pain medicine because he doesn't like to take medicine and it made him feel light-headed and groggy. He indicates that he will just have to "tough it out." Questions to consider:

· How would you approach this situation?
· Do you think the patient will receive the full benefit of his therapy sessions if he is limited by pain?
· How could evidence be incorporated into this scenario?

Introduction

In this chapter, we will discuss the importance of integrating patient values and circumstances into the evidence based decision-making process. In Chapter 2, we reviewed Sackett's definition of evidence based practice: "the integration of the best available research evidence with the clinician's expertise and the patient's individual values and circumstances."[1] The clinician needs to understand the meaning of patient values and patient circumstances (Fig. 3.1). **Patient values** can be defined as the preferences that a patient and family bring to a patient care interaction. The patient's and family's preferences may be based on cultural or religious expectations, personal attitudes and beliefs, life experiences and learning, or most likely a combination of these factors. **Patient circumstances** can be defined as the current environment or situation of the patient. This could refer to a patient's living situation, family or social situation, or resources available to provide care and manage daily living tasks.[2] An additional consideration is the health literacy of the patient and/or family members. **Health literacy** has been defined as "the degree to which individuals have the capacity to obtain, process, and understand basic health information and services needed to make appropriate health decisions."[3] Health-care providers must ensure that patients understand the information being provided to them.

Health Literacy

Health literacy can have a major impact on a patient's health. Limited health literacy is associated with poor health. Research has shown that individuals with limited health literacy have the following characteristics:

- They are less likely to use preventive care.
- They enter the health-care system when they are sicker.

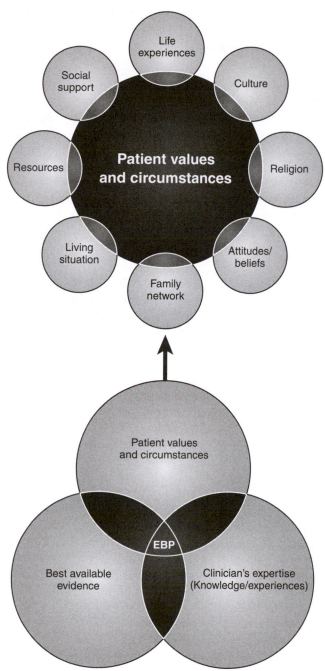

Figure 3.1 Patient values and circumstances are one of the three components of evidence based practice. A variety of factors contribute to patient values and circumstances.

- They have a higher rate of preventable hospitalizations and use of emergency services.
- They are more likely to have chronic conditions but are less able to effectively manage those conditions.[4]

Patients must be able to understand why an intervention or medication is important and how it will affect their life and their health. For example, a patient may stop taking a blood pressure medication when she feels okay or has a normal blood pressure reading if she doesn't understand that the medication must be taken routinely in order to be effective. A clinician must be able to explain how the medication works, why it is important, and potential risks of noncompliance in words that a patient can clearly understand. A patient may stop doing a home exercise program because "the exercises made me sore" if he doesn't understand that muscle soreness is a normal response to a strength training program. The clinician must be able to explain the purpose of the home exercise program, the importance of improving strength, and potential health risks of noncompliance in language that is clear, concise, and easy to understand.

Communication is critical to improving an individual's health literacy and should incorporate plain language. **Plain language** can be defined as clear, straightforward expression that uses as few words as possible to convey a message.[5] Plain language conveys a grammatically correct, accurate, and concise message in a professional manner. It can be easily understood by your patient and involves using simple language, defining medical or technical terms, organizing information so that the most important information comes first, and breaking complicated information into "bite-sized" chunks.[6] The U.S. government has made efforts to ensure that all government documents are written in plain language (Fig. 3.2). The most recent government mandate, the Plain

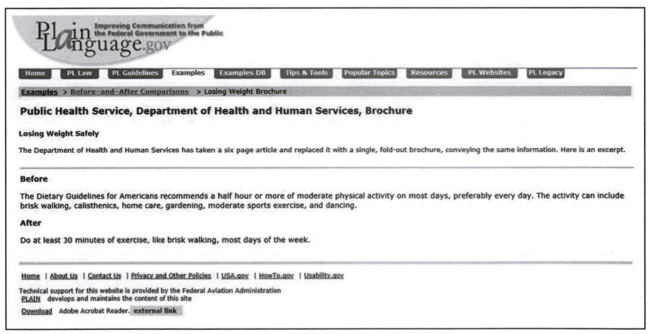

Figure 3.2 Plain language is clear, straightforward expression that uses as few words as possible to convey a message. This example from www.plainlanguage.gov demonstrates the concept of plain language. *Source:* Screenshot from Plain Language.gov (www.plainlanguage.gov), the Plain Language Action and Information Network. Accessed January 23, 2015.

Language Act of 2010, requires government agencies to write in plain language. This includes all government health-care agencies, including the Centers for Medicare and Medicaid Services and the National Institutes of Health. Clinicians can access numerous resources addressing plain language at the following websites:

- www.plainlanguage.gov
- www.nih.gov
- www.health.gov

Health literacy can be affected by a variety of factors and circumstances. Some patients may have been exposed to a long history of conventional wisdom and "old wives' tales" regarding health issues and health remedies. This can make it more difficult to educate a patient about current health problems and best evidence related to treatment. A patient's educational level or reading level should dictate how information is presented. Patients with specific diagnoses that affect cognition will likely require different strategies for communication. An individual who is confronted by a major illness or injury might become overwhelmed and unable to process information as well as under normal circumstances. Can you recall a time when you received information from a health-care provider that was difficult to understand? If so, think about how the information might have been provided more effectively.

Learning Task

Access one of the websites listed earlier to complete this task. Using resources found on the website, translate the following statement into plain language:

Diabetes mellitus symptoms include polyuria, polydipsia, and polyphagia. A diagnosis of diabetes mellitus requires frequent blood glucose testing to avoid hypoglycemic or hyperglycemic episodes and prevent complications such as ketoacidosis and diabetic coma. Chronic diabetes mellitus complications include diabetic retinopathy, cardiovascular disease, peripheral vascular disease, cerebrovascular accident, diabetic neuropathy, and renal failure.

Patient-Centered Care and Shared Decision-Making

For centuries, health care has primarily followed a traditional, or physician-centered, model, which involved a physician or health-care provider making treatment decisions for a patient. This model was geared toward a health-care provider telling a patient, "This is what you need to do." Patients were frequently viewed as passive consumers of health care. In more recent years, health care has begun to shift focus from the health-care provider to the individual patient. In **patient-centered care**, patients actively participate in their own health care, and the patient and family are the center of care. Patients determine the services received based on their own needs and preferences and the recommendations of health-care providers. This model is geared more toward a health-care provider telling a patient, "These are your options—what would you like to do?" The patient-centered model is sometimes called the patient- and family-centered model because the family is often involved in the decision-making process as well as the patient.[7] A key concept of patient-centered care is that health-care providers honor patient and family perspectives and choices. Health-care providers must provide unbiased information to patients and encourage patients and families to participate in making decisions.

Shared decision-making, which is a component of patient-centered care, places an emphasis on the collaboration between patients and health-care providers. Shared decision-making can be defined as "a collaborative process that allows patients and their providers to make health care decisions together, taking into account the best scientific evidence available as well as the patient's values and preferences."[8] You may notice that this definition includes the same key elements as the definition of evidence based practice: best available evidence, provider's clinical experience, and the patient's values. This approach to decision-making can be particularly useful when there is more than one clinically appropriate treatment option and not necessarily a best option. Patients who have taken an active role in treatment decisions are more satisfied with their care and have a more positive outlook about their health situation.[7] Older patients may have more difficulty with shared decision-making if they are accustomed to the more traditional model of care. However, a clinician should make every effort to involve the patient in decision-making related to goals, outcomes, and interventions.

Obligations of Care

Providing individuals with good health care should be a primary goal of health-care providers and health-care organizations. A basic underlying principle in health care is "first do no harm." Today's health-care professionals are held to a much higher standard than doing no harm, however. The American Physical Therapy Association has outlined ethical standards and core values for members of the profession.[9] The core values of the profession are accountability, altruism, compassion/caring, excellence, integrity, professional duty, and social responsibility. The Code of Ethics for physical therapists and the Standards of Ethical Conduct for physical therapist assistants (PTAs) are based in large part on the core values and outline the ethical obligations of clinicians. These ethical obligations include respecting the inherent dignity and rights of all individuals, being trustworthy and compassionate in addressing patient needs and rights, demonstrating integrity in relationships with patients and families, and being accountable for making sound judgments. Box 3.1 provides a summary of the Standards of Ethical Conduct for PTAs.

Box 3.1 | American Physical Therapy Association Standards of Ethical Conduct for Physical Therapist Assistants

---

Physical therapist assistants shall:
- Respect the inherent dignity and rights of all individuals.
- Be trustworthy and compassionate in addressing the rights and needs of patients/clients.
- Make sound decisions in collaboration with the physical therapist and within the boundaries established by laws and regulations.
- Demonstrate integrity in their relationships with patient/clients, families, colleagues, students, other health-care providers, employers, payers, and the public.
- Fulfill their legal and ethical obligations.
- Enhance their competence through the lifelong acquisition and refinement of knowledge, skills, and abilities.
- Support organizational behaviors and business practices that benefit patients/clients and society.
- Participate in efforts to meet the health needs of people locally, nationally, or globally.

Source: www.apta.org/uploadedFiles/APTAorg/About_Us/Policies/Ethics/StandardsEthical ConductPTA.pdf. Accessed June 30, 2015.

Patients have certain rights that have been established through federal and state laws. In addition, many health-care facilities have a patient bill of rights. Clinicians should make sure that their patients are informed about and understand their rights as patients. A key patient right is the right to participate in treatment decisions. Patients have the right to know all of their treatment options, and they have the right to participate in decisions about their care. The American Medical Association has indicated that "the patient's right of self-decision can be effectively exercised only if the patient possesses enough information to enable an intelligent choice."[10] The American Physical Therapy Association ethical guidelines include an expectation that the clinician must respect the patient's right to make decisions and must communicate findings to the patients.[9] Patients have the right to designate someone to participate in health-care decisions if they become unable to make their own decisions.

A key patient right that is necessary for a patient to participate in treatment decisions is informed consent. **Informed consent** can be defined as the process by which the clinician discloses appropriate information to a competent patient so that the patient can make a voluntary choice to accept or refuse treatment.[9-11] The World Confederation of Physical Therapists Declaration of Principle on Informed Consent stipulates that informed consent must include clear and adequate information about the following:

- The treatment to be provided
- Explanation of risks that may be associated with the treatment
- Potential and expected benefits of treatment
- Anticipated timeframes and costs
- Reasonable alternatives to treatment[11]

The information provided should be presented in plain language, and the clinician must ensure that the patient understands and has an opportunity to ask questions or clarify. In addition, the clinician should ensure that the patient is competent to make an informed decision. This may be difficult at times but is critical to informed consent. The final component of informed consent is patient acceptance. The clinician should make sure that the patient has agreed to the treatment before proceeding.

Patient Values and Circumstances

Every individual has a unique set of values and preferences that he or she uses to make decisions. An individual's values and preferences are molded by society, by the individual's culture, by religion or absence of religion, by life experiences (both positive and negative), and by knowledge and learning. Throughout life, that individual will be placed in ever-changing circumstances that will also affect decisions. Let's imagine the following scenario:

You slipped and fell on a patch of ice and broke your right wrist. The emergency department physician calls in an orthopedic surgeon, who provides you with two options: (1) align the bones with a cast (alignment may not be ideal) and allow to heal, or (2) perform surgery to repair the fracture and ensure good alignment. The surgery is expensive but will allow a shorter healing time.

Now let's look at some different patient circumstances that might affect health care.

- You are a college student who is still covered by your parent's insurance. You have a number of friends who are more than happy to help you with tasks while you recover and help you keep up with assignments. You are left-handed, so you will still be able to write, use your computer, and perform other tasks without using your right hand.

- You are a 38-year-old man who is currently unemployed and living in your car. You do not have any insurance or financial resources. You try to pick up some odd jobs, mostly manual labor, as often as you can to make a little money for food and gas. You are right-handed so you are concerned about not being able to work.
- You are a 43-year-old executive who has excellent health-care coverage and accumulated sick leave. You have a housekeeper at home to do household chores and help with your children. You are left-handed, and you have an administrative assistant who can do most of your writing, keyboarding, and other tasks when you return to work.
- You are an 84-year-old woman living alone on a small farm outside of town. You have been able to take care of yourself and your home without any help, but it has been getting more difficult. You have no family nearby, and most of your friends are no longer living. Your only income is Social Security and a small monthly annuity payment. You have Medicare insurance. You are right-handed.

These individuals would likely make different decisions regarding whether to have surgery or not, based on a variety of factors. They also might make different decisions regarding discharge plans when they leave the hospital. Those individuals who have insurance might be more likely to decide to have surgery. Someone with no insurance and no financial resources might opt to have the wrist casted. Someone who lives alone would likely need to stay somewhere else after leaving the hospital, such as a rehabilitation or skilled nursing facility. Culture and religion are also factors in making health-care decisions. In some cultures, older family members are revered and taken care of by younger family members. Some religions adhere to faith healing and do not advocate surgery.

How do we find out about a patient's values and circumstances? This is typically accomplished by gathering information during the history portion of the initial examination by the clinician, but important information can also be collected during follow-up visits. Patients or family members may have forgotten to mention a key piece of information, such as a recent onset of falling. If a patient is not able to provide a history, the clinician will need to speak with a family member or friend or review past medical records to gather the information. Open communication is critical to gathering information from patient and family as well as collaborating in making health-care decisions. As stated previously, the clinician is obligated to respect the rights and dignity of all patients. When patients are participating in making health-care decisions, the clinician needs to understand the factors that are affecting the patient's decision. Although something may not seem significant to you as a clinician, if it is important to the patient, then it is important in his or her plan of care.

SUMMARY

The three key components of evidence based practice include the best available research evidence, the clinician's expertise, and the patient's values and circumstances. Health literacy, which refers to the patient's ability to understand basic health information necessary to make appropriate health decisions, is a key component in the overall health of individuals. In recent years, health care has been moving from a traditional model to a patient-centered care model. This model places the patient and family at the center of care. Shared decision-making is a component of patient-centered care and includes the collaboration between the patient and the clinician in making informed health-care decisions. Health-care professionals have ethical and legal obligations for providing care and must respect a patient's right to participate in making decisions. Patients also have rights, and the clinician should ensure that patients understand their rights and responsibilities within the health-care system. Informed consent is an important part of the communication between the clinician and the patient and is required for a patient to be able to make an informed decision about health-care options. Patient values and circumstances affect health-care decisions, and clinicians should respect patient preferences when determining a plan of care.

● Case Scenario

You are a PTA providing home care in a small city, and you recently began treating a 71-year-old woman who was seen in the emergency department following a fall. She hit her head and her right shoulder when she fell, but x-rays revealed no fractures or other significant injuries. Her primary care physician referred her for home health physical therapy to address her deconditioned state and her balance. After several visits, you notice that dishes and trash are piling up, and the house was already cluttered and full of furniture, newspapers, magazines, and boxes. You also notice that the patient is wearing dirty clothes and her hair is unkempt. The patient has always taken pride in being a strong, independent woman. She has told you that she raised four sons by herself after her husband died at an early age and that her sons are now all successful businessmen living with their families in other parts of the country. She refused the services of a home health aide because she said she could take care of herself. You become concerned that she is not able to adequately care for herself, and you are also concerned that even if her balance improves, she is at risk for falling because of the clutter in the home.

CASE QUESTIONS

1. How would you approach this situation?

_____

_____

2. What information would you need to share with the therapist who is directing her care?

_____

_____

3. What are some possible options that might be presented to the patient to help with her situation?

_____

_____

Learning Task
Using any resources available, identify an organization in your community that provides assistance to elderly people. Gather information (e.g., websites, brochures) and be prepared to participate in group discussion with classmates to address the case scenario.

Review Activities

1. In your own words, define (a) patient values and (b) patient circumstances.

_____

_____

_____

_____

2. Briefly explain the importance of health literacy.

_____

_____

_____

_____

3. Provide an example of using plain language in place of a medical term.

_____

_____

_____

_____

4. Identify who should be involved in shared decision-making.

_____

_____

_____

_____

5. List the types of information that must be included in informed consent.

_____

_____

_____

_____

MATCHING

_____ 1. Informed consent   A. Current situation of a patient

_____ 2. Plain language   B. Collaborative process of making
                                         health-care decisions

_____ 3. Shared decision-making

C. Ability of individual to understand basic health information

_____ 4. Patient values

D. Clinician discloses adequate information for patient to make voluntary decision

_____ 5. Patient circumstances

E. Clear information using few words to convey message

_____ 6. Health literacy

F. Preferences of a patient based on expectations and beliefs

▨ References

1. Sackett DL. Evidence-based medicine. _Semin Perinatol._ 1997;21(1):3-5.
2. Hack LM, Gwyer J. _Evidence Into Practice: Integrating Judgment, Values, and Research._ Philadelphia, PA: FA Davis; 2013.
3. U.S. Department of Health and Human Services. Health Communication, Health Literacy and e-Health. www.health.gov. Accessed June 30, 2015.
4. Institute of Education Sciences. The health literacy of America's adults: results from the 2003 National Assessment of Adult Literacy. http://nces.ed.gov. Accessed June 30, 2015.
5. Federal Plain Language Guidelines. Plain Language website. www.plainlanguage.gov. Accessed June 30, 2015.
6. National Institutes of Health. Clear communication: health literacy. www.nih.gov. Accessed June 30, 2015.
7. Agency for Healthcare Research and Quality. Expanding patient-centered care to empower patients and assist providers and shared decision making. www.ahrq.gov. Accessed June 30, 2015.
8. Informed Medical Decisions Foundation. What is shared decision making? www.informedmedicaldecisions.org. Accessed June 30, 2015.
9. American Physical Therapy Association. www.apta.org. Accessed June 30, 2015.
10. American Medical Association. www.ama.org. Accessed June 30, 2015.
11. Bennett J. Liability awareness: informed consent—tips and caveats for PTs. _PT in Motion._ December 2007.

Part Two provides an abridged discussion of research concepts and the different types of research likely to be encountered in a search for best available evidence. Chapter 4 provides an introduction to basic research terminology, including sampling, validity, reliability, and research design. The chapter will prepare the reader to study and understand Chapters 5 to 8. Chapter 5 illustrates the basic concepts of experimental research, including randomized controlled trials (RCTs) and quasi-experimental designs. The chapter will explain the importance of experimental research in expanding the physical therapy body of evidence. Chapter 6 describes the basic concepts of exploratory research, including cohort studies, predictive research, and methodological/reliability and validity studies. The chapter includes a comparison of exploratory research to other types of research and discusses the rationale for exploratory research. Chapter 7 discusses various types of descriptive research, including normative studies, qualitative research, and case studies. Descriptive research often provides a basis for further investigation. Chapter 8 discusses systematic reviews, meta-analyses, and clinical practice guidelines. The role of these types of sources in synthesizing a growing body of evidence will be explored.

The overall goal of Part Two is to acquaint the physical therapist assistant (PTA) with research and common research terminology. It will also assist in preparing the PTA to participate in evidence based practice. The role of the PTA in utilizing various types of evidence as part of a physical therapist (PT)/PTA team will be emphasized. Examples of research are provided throughout the chapters to facilitate the reader's understanding.

- Chapter 4: Research Terminology
- Chapter 5: Experimental Research
- Chapter 6: Exploratory Research
- Chapter 7: Descriptive Research
- Chapter 8: Research Reviews and Clinical Practice Guidelines

Research Terminology

Chapter at a Glance

Learning Outcomes

After reading this chapter, the reader will be able to:

· Describe the differences between reliability and validity.
· List examples of types of reliability and validity commonly discussed in physical therapy research.
· Discuss the concept of bias in research.
· Differentiate between population and sample and describe how they are related.
· Explain the concept of generalization.
· Identify key differences between probability and nonprobability sampling and provide examples.
· Define key terminology related to research design.
· Describe the distinguishing characteristics of research design categories.

Key Terms

· Accessible population
· Bias
· Comparison group
· Dependent variable
· Descriptive research
· Experimental research
· Exploratory research
· Generalization
· Independent variable
· Methodological research
· Nonprobability sampling
· Normative research
· Placebo
· Population of interest
· Probability sampling
· Prospective
· Publication bias
· Qualitative research
· Quantitative research
· Random assignment
· Random selection
· Reliability
· Retrospective
· Sample
· Sampling bias
· Validity
· Variable

◘ FOOD FOR THOUGHT

You are a physical therapist assistant in a large teaching hospital. During the monthly staff meeting, the Director of Rehabilitation describes a research study being developed by a group of researchers in the hospital that will involve the physical therapy department. The study will be investigating two different surgical procedures for lumbar laminectomy: a standard procedure and a new procedure developed by a group of surgeons in Boston. The therapy department will be responsible for taking some measurements 2 days after surgery, including a functional mobility scale.

Questions to consider:
· What type of individuals would be chosen for the study?
· Do you think this would be considered an experimental study?
· Would it be important for all of the therapists to take the measurements using the same technique?

Introduction

Research studies may be conducted for a variety of reasons. Some studies are designed to investigate cause and effect. Other studies are designed to investigate relationships between variables. Studies may also be designed to describe characteristics of a population. The type of research study and the research design will be determined by the research question being asked. Before beginning a discussion of research design, however, some key terms will be introduced. The terminology in this chapter will apply to all types of research discussed in the following chapters. A considerable amount of information is presented in this chapter in order to frame the discussions in the following chapters. Therefore, the readers are encouraged to read and review any sections that they find difficult to understand.

Reliability

Reliability is defined as the ability to produce the same results in repeated measures when the conditions are the same.[1] Reliability primarily refers to tests and measurements. For example, if you assess a patient's strength and a colleague assesses the same patient's strength, you should both get the same score. Statistical analysis of reliability is typically conducted using a test of correlation, or relationship. A test of correlation will compare test results to determine how closely related the scores are to each other. The most commonly reported statistical test for reliability is the intraclass correlation coefficient, or ICC. The ICC provides a measurement of both correlation and agreement and ranges from 0.0 to 1.0. A perfect correlation/agreement would be a 1.0, and no correlation/agreement would be reported as 0.0. Therefore, a higher score indicates greater reliability of the tool. Table 4.1 provides examples of different types of reliability that are commonly seen in physical therapy research.

Research articles should address reliability for any tests or measures used in the study. Threats to reliability include the following:

- *Multiple data collectors:* If multiple data collectors are utilized in a study, did they all have the same level of expertise in the testing procedure? Did they receive the same level of training in the testing procedure?
- *Recording materials:* Are all data metrics being recorded in the same manner? Were metrics recorded using the same methods?

Table 4.1 | Examples of Types of Reliability Commonly Seen in Physical Therapy Research Literature

Type of Reliability*	Definition	Additional Comments	Example
Test-retest	Establishes whether a measurement tool can measure a variable consistently	A small number of subjects are tested on two different occasions with conditions being as identical as possible; commonly seen with measurement tools that are self-reported by the subject	In a study investigating patient's fear of falling, the measurement tool could be administered on two consecutive visits; the test results are then compared
Intrarater	Establishes whether a rater can consistently conduct a test and record results	A rater will conduct the same test multiple times, with short intervals between tests, on a small number of subjects; it can be difficult to separate test-retest and intrarater reliability for tests that are administered rather than self-reported	In a study examining a patient's balance, the rater could administer a balance assessment on two or three consecutive mornings or one morning and the same afternoon
Interrater	Establishes whether multiple raters can consistently conduct a test and record results	More than one rater will administer a test on the same subjects within a short period of time, ideally at the same session; for tools that require observation only, both raters should observe at the same time	In a study investigating the quality of a patient's gait, two raters could observe a subject carrying out the assigned tasks, with each rater recording the results independently

- *Environment:* Circumstances at the time of the data collection may affect data collection, such as time of day, temperature, and floor surface.
- *Participants:* Factors such as fatigue, hunger, or stress can affect measurements, particularly with repeated measures.

Validity

Validity is traditionally defined as the soundness or accuracy of a conclusion or measurement.[2] The term *validity* can be used in relation to a test to describe whether the test actually measures what it is supposed to measure.[1] For example, you will likely be taught how to use a universal goniometer to measure joint range of motion—does this instrument actually measure the motion of the joint? The term *validity* can also be used in relation to a research study. Hack and Gwyer define this type of validity as trustworthiness.[3] In other words: Can you trust the results of the research study, or is the study untrustworthy in some way? If a researcher selects participants for a study with the greatest potential for a good outcome and does not include individuals with less potential, will the results be valid? Think about a researcher who has designed a study to investigate the effectiveness of a new treatment and plans to utilize a placebo group for comparison. A **placebo** is defined as a harmless medication or procedure that has no therapeutic effect and is used as a comparison to an experimental medication or procedure; the placebo group would reasonably be expected to show no improvement. If the researcher placed younger, healthier subjects in the treatment group and older, less healthy subjects in the placebo group, do you think the results would be trustworthy?

Types of validity can be divided broadly into external validity and internal validity. External validity deals with the similarity of the people in the study to the entire population of interest and will be discussed further in the section on sampling. Methods used by the researcher in selecting a sample for a study affect external validity. Internal validity deals with the research procedures used to control for other possible explanations for the outcomes of the study. Some types of validity are assessed by subjective means only (face, content). Other types of validity are assessed using a correlation coefficient (criterion related). Table 4.2 provides examples of types of validity commonly seen in physical therapy research.

Threats to validity include factors such as the following:

- *History:* Did an unexpected event outside of the study occur during the testing period that might have affected the results? An example would be a study investigating strength improvement in high school athletes based on an exercise protocol. If the majority of subjects began off-season training at their school during the testing period, the results would be affected.
- *Maturation of subjects:* Did changes occur because of normal developmental changes of subjects in the study? If a study lasts several years, it is likely that subjects would experience improvement in performance regardless of the study protocol.
- *Selection:* With subjects being assigned to different groups, were the selected groups equal at the beginning of the testing period? If subjects are added to a study over a period of time, it might be difficult to determine whether groups are equal until the end of the testing period. The method for assigning subjects to groups would affect the likelihood that the groups are equal.
- *Experimental mortality:* Did more subjects drop out of one group than another group? Did subjects who dropped out of the study affect the results of the study?
- *Testing:* If a pre-test was administered, did it affect the scores of the post-test? In other words, if the same test is used for pre- and post-testing, subject responses on the post-test may be affected by previous exposure to the questions.

Table 4.2 | Examples of Types of Validity Commonly Seen in Physical Therapy Research Literature

Type of Validity*	Definition	Additional Comments	Example
Face	Establishes that an instrument appears to measure what it is supposed to measure	Face validity is subjective and the weakest form of validity; it should be reported if no other type of validity is possible	In a study investigating patient's fear of falling, the questions on the measurement tool must clearly ask questions related to falling and fear of falling
Content	Establishes that an instrument covers all critical aspects of a variable being tested	Content validity is subjective and is determined based on the research question—in other words, what is the researcher attempting to measure?	In a study examining a patient's balance, the measurement tool should cover all aspects of balance as defined by the research question
Criterion-related	Establishes that an instrument is valid based on comparison to a gold standard test	Criterion-related validity is objective and is determined by identifying whether the new test results correlate with results from the gold standard; can also be determined by identifying whether the new test result can predict the results on the gold standard test	In a study investigating the quality of a patient's gait, the new test and the gold standard test must both be measuring the same aspects of gait quality, and would both be conducted on each subject to compare the results

- *Measurement:* Were all subjects measured in the same way? Were instruments used for measurement calibrated for accuracy?
- *Contamination:* Did subjects in the control group know what type of treatment the experimental group was receiving? If so, did that affect the results?

Figure 4.1 depicts the relationship between reliability and validity. Examples of reliability and validity issues will be discussed in the following chapters.

Learning Task
Using any search tool available, locate an article of interest that uses a measurement instrument/scale or describes the development of a measurement tool. Read the article and find discussions about reliability and validity. Did all of the articles provide a discussion about reliability? Validity? What different types of reliability and validity were discussed in the article? Be prepared to discuss your findings with your classmates.

Bias

Clinicians should have a good understanding of the term bias because it will be encountered when reviewing and appraising research articles. **Bias** can generally be defined as "any tendency which prevents unprejudiced consideration of a question."[4] In research, the term *bias* can be used in a variety of ways. Bias can be due to errors in

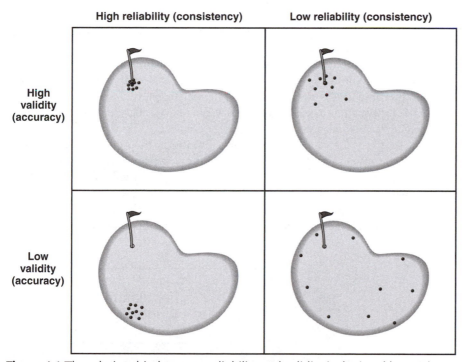

Figure 4.1 The relationship between reliability and validity is depicted here. The area represents a golf course green, and the hole with the flag is the object, or target. The black dots represent 10 golf balls hit onto the green. When reliability is high, the golf balls are clustered, showing consistency. When validity is high, the golf balls are close to the target, showing accuracy. When both reliability and validity are high, the golf balls are clustered close to the target.

sampling from a population, or it can be due to using an incorrect statistical test. Bias can also be due to actions by the investigator, intentional or not, that influence the outcomes. Bias can occur at any phase of research: planning, data collection, analysis, and even publication. The most common bias encountered during the publication phase is publication bias. **Publication bias** can be defined as the decreased likelihood of publication for research with negative or nonsignificant results compared with research with positive results. Investigators may be less likely to submit a research report for publication if the results are not significant or show negative results. Journals may be less likely to accept reports of studies with results that are negative or not significant. Bias will be discussed throughout the following chapters as well as strategies to reduce or overcome bias.

Populations and Samples

One of the first questions to ask about a study is, "What is the population of interest?" Let's assume that a researcher wants to conduct a study to determine which type of therapeutic exercise is most effective in increasing hip strength in patients following a bipolar hemiarthroplasty. The best way to determine which type of exercise is most effective would be to study the entire population of interest. A **population of interest,** or target population, is the group of individuals who meet a specific set of criteria (Fig. 4.2). The population of interest in our example would be all patients everywhere who have undergone a bipolar hemiarthroplasty. Obviously it would be impossible in this case for a researcher to study the entire population in terms of access, time, and costs. The researcher will therefore need to identify an accessible population. The **accessible population** is the actual group of subjects available to be selected for the study, such as patients who have undergone a bipolar hemiarthroplasty in a local medical center. This accessible population is likely still too large for each individual to participate in the study, so a sample can be selected. A **sample** is a subset of a population selected for a study. The sample should have the same characteristics and variability as the larger group. In our example, the researcher will select a sample from the patients of the local medical center who have undergone a bipolar hemiarthroplasty. Using a sample allows a researcher to investigate a research question with a manageable number of individuals, thus reducing costs and time.[5]

For the results of the study to be generalized to the entire population, the method in which the sample is selected is important. **Generalization** means that the results of a study conducted on a sample can reasonably be applied more broadly to all individuals within the population.[1] How can the responses of a small group of subjects be generalized to a population with confidence? The answer lies in the sampling procedures used, which can minimize the level of sampling bias. **Sampling bias** is the

Figure 4.2 For sampling, a researcher must define the population of interest and identify the portion of the population of interest that is accessible. A sample will be selected from the accessible population.

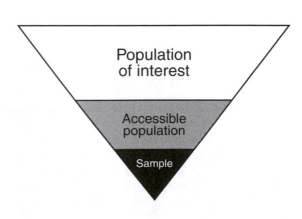

Population of interest

Accessible population

Sample

over- or under-representation of certain characteristics of the population within the sample. For example, imagine that you want to investigate the opinions of young adults about healthy lifestyle behaviors. Your sample is drawn from students at a local university. Do you think the outcomes of such a study could be generalized to the population of all young adults? What about young adults who serve in the military, or young adults who cannot afford to go to college and are working full-time? Is it likely that their opinions might be different from students at a university? The study could provide valuable information but could not readily be generalized to the entire population of young adults.

Researchers can use a variety of methods to select a sample from the accessible population. Methods of sampling can be categorized as probability sampling or nonprobability sampling. The key difference between the two categories of sampling is random selection. **Random selection** is defined as a method of selection in which every individual within the population has an equal chance of being selected for the sample.[1,5,6] **Probability sampling** uses random selection and is most likely to result in a sample that truly represents the population. **Nonprobability sampling** uses a method of sampling that is not random, so individuals within the population do not all have the same chance of being selected.[5,6] Therefore the sample is less likely to have the same characteristics as the population. Table 4.3 provides a comparison and examples of probability and nonprobability sampling. Examples of probability and nonprobability sampling are described next, but the reader should understand that a wide variety of sampling methods exist.

Probability Sampling

Simple Random Sampling

Simple random sampling (Fig. 4.3) requires that the researcher has access to each individual within the population in some way, such as a list of names. As an example, let's assume that the population of interest for a study is all students currently enrolled in a PTA program in Texas, and the sample will include 75 students. The researcher could obtain a list of students from all of the programs, place each name in a bowl, mix them up, and draw names at random until 75 names were drawn. The researcher could also choose to use a computer program to randomly select 75 names from the full list. Either of these would result in a random sample derived from the population of interest.[1]

Table 4.3 | A Comparison of Probability and Nonprobability Sampling Methods

	Probability	Nonprobability
Is random selection used?	Yes	No
Can results be generalized to entire population?	More likely	Less likely
Is there a sampling bias?	Less likely	More likely
Examples	Simple random	Stratified random
	Cluster	Convenience
	Purposive	Snowball

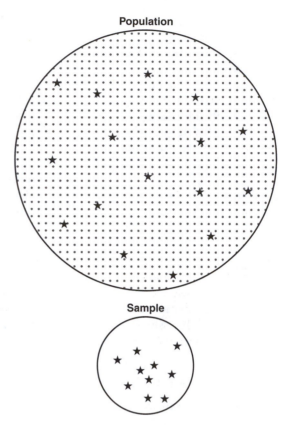

Figure 4.3 Simple random sampling occurs when researchers have access to the entire population and use a random method of selection. As depicted in the figure, the entire population is represented by dots, whereas the individuals randomly selected are depicted by stars. With simple random sampling, the selected subjects should be randomly distributed throughout the population.

Stratified Random Sampling

Stratified random sampling (Fig. 4.4) can be used when an investigator wants to ensure adequate representation from subgroups within the population. Members of the population are placed into subsets based on specific relevant characteristics that are not overlapping.[5] Using the previous example of PTA students in the state of Texas, the investigator might divide the students into groups based on ethnicity, gender, or age. The characteristic chosen for forming subsets, or strata, must be relevant to the variables of interest for the study. The investigator then obtains a random sample from each of the subsets. This method is useful when the investigator wants to make sure that a key subgroup, particularly a minority group, is accurately represented in the sample. The investigator may be interested in support services utilized by students during the course of the PTA program. The investigator wants to ensure that older students, who typically make up a small percentage of PTA students, are well represented. A decision could be made to divide the students into age groups before choosing the sample, then randomly select a specified number of subjects from each age group. This method would ensure that older students are well represented.

Cluster Sampling

Cluster sampling (Fig. 4.5) is a method of sampling that can be used when a population is so large and so geographically diverse that it is not possible to obtain a list of the entire population.[1] As an example, an investigator wants to conduct a study involving physical therapists in Texas who practice in public school settings. Imagine the time and effort it would require to obtain an accurate list of all therapists in this population. With cluster sampling, the researcher could choose a random sample of five counties

Population by age

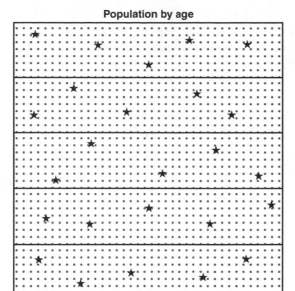

Sample

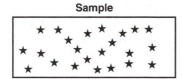

Figure 4.4 Stratified random sampling can be used to ensure adequate representation from subgroups within a population. The population is stratified based on relevant characteristics (e.g., age) before subjects are randomly selected.

Population

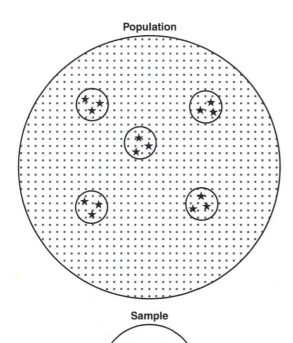

Sample

Figure 4.5 Cluster sampling can be used when it is difficult or impossible to access the entire population. The researcher can choose a random sample of locations, then select a random sample of subjects at each location.

in Texas (a list of counties is readily available), then randomly select five public school settings in each county (lists of public schools are also easily available). The researcher would then be able to conduct a study with a sample of physical therapists practicing in those randomly selected 25 public schools. This provides a much more manageable group of subjects but may also result in a sample that does not accurately reflect the population. The sample is more likely to be representative if the study uses the largest sample possible.

Nonprobability Sampling

Nonprobability sampling is often used in real life because it is typically difficult to get a true random sample. Nonprobability sampling can be accomplished in several different ways.

Convenience Sampling

The most commonly used method of nonprobability sampling is convenience, or accidental, sampling (Fig. 4.6). This method chooses subjects based on availability and results in a sample that most likely does not represent the population of interest.[3] An example of convenience sampling would be recruiting volunteers for a study. The researcher may post flyers on bulletin boards in college buildings or physical therapy clinics identifying the criteria for the study and asking for volunteers. In this case, the sample would only include subjects who took the initiative to respond to the flyer. A researcher may also choose to recruit all patients entering a physical therapy clinic during a specified period of time who meet the criteria for a study. For example, a researcher decides to conduct a study involving patients who have recently (within the past year) been

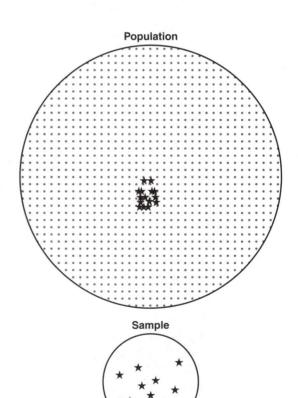

Figure 4.6 Convenience sampling chooses subjects based on availability, typically by location. With convenience sampling, the selected subjects are from one area of the population and do not necessarily represent the population.

diagnosed with a stroke. For a defined period of time, all new patients who were recently diagnosed with a stroke will be recruited for the study and can choose or decline to participate.

Purposive Sampling

Purposive sampling (Fig. 4.7) methodology requires the researcher to select specific subjects for a study based on specific criteria.[5] Although it is similar to convenience sampling, purposive sampling goes beyond availability to selection based on a specific characteristic within the population of interest. Building on the previous example, a researcher may decide to study the impact of a recent stroke (within the past year) on a patient's marriage. In this instance, the researcher might interview all new patients who were recently diagnosed with a stroke but will select only those patients with a living spouse for the study. As another example, you might have encountered someone outside a store or mall who approached you to ask you a few questions. This individual was likely using purposive sampling—you may have been approached because you just left a particular store, purchased a particular product, or looked as though you were within a certain age group.

Snowball Sampling

The snowball sampling (Fig. 4.8) methodology involves identifying individuals who meet the criteria for the study, then asking them to identify others who also meet the criteria.[2] The researcher will then contact those individuals to recruit for the study. This process would continue until an adequate sample size was obtained. This method of sampling is most useful when the target population is difficult to find, such as homeless individuals, or when the purpose of the study includes sensitive topics, such as drug use or eating disorders.

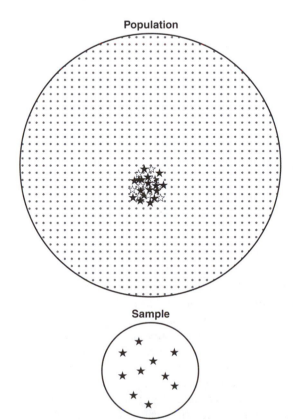

Figure 4.7 Purposive sampling chooses subjects based on availability and a specified characteristic. If the researcher is interested in individuals between the ages of 18 and 24 years, a number of individuals may be considered, but only those within the desired age range are selected. Dark stars represent individuals within the desired age range, whereas the light stars represent individuals who fell outside of the 18- to 24-year age range and were not selected.

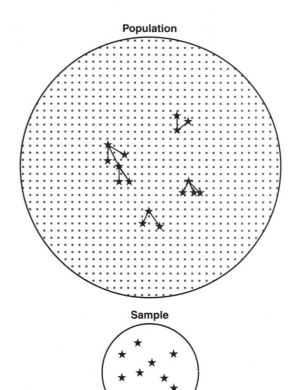

Figure 4.8 Snowball sampling chooses subjects based on specific criteria. Those subjects will be asked to identify others who also meet the criteria. The process continues until an adequate sample is obtained.

Learning Task

Using the article you found that addressed a measurement scale, find the section that discusses the population of interest and the selection of subjects.

• Does the article identify the population of interest? The type of sampling?

• Would the sampling method be classified as probability or nonprobability?

• If the specific sampling method was not identified, can you categorize it (i.e., cluster, convenience, snowball)?

• Discuss with your classmates to determine the variety of sampling methods found.

Research Design

Research design is the overall structure or framework of an experiment. The research design will depend on the purpose of the study and the type of research question being asked (Table 4.4). The design will determine the methods and procedures used, including how participants will be selected, how data will be collected, what instruments will be used and how they will be used, and how data will be analyzed. Studies that investigate cause and effect are categorized as experimental. Studies that investigate relationships between variables are categorized as exploratory. A third category, descriptive, includes studies that describe attributes of a population.

Before continuing the discussion of types of research design, it will be important to define another term commonly used in research—*variables*. Portney and Watkins

Table 4.4 | Types of Research Designs Listed by Category

	Category	Purpose Types
Experimental	Determine cause and effect	True experimental design
		Quasi-experimental design
Exploratory	Determine relationships	Cohort studies
		Correlational research
		Predictive research
		Methodological research
Descriptive	Describe populations	Qualitative research
		Normative research
		Descriptive surveys
		Case studies

define a **variable** as a characteristic that can be manipulated or observed and can take on different values.[2] Two types of variables are commonly identified in research articles. The **independent variable** is the variable being controlled by the researcher.[1] The **dependent variable** is the variable being measured as an outcome. For example, in a study investigating the effect of a new exercise protocol, the exercise protocol is the independent variable. The dependent variable might be strength, or it might be flexibility or balance. The investigator is looking to see if the dependent variable changes as the independent variable is adjusted. It is not unusual for a study to include more than one dependent variable. A study investigating the impact of beginning therapy the day of surgery following total hip replacement might use dependent variables of hospital length of stay, patient's pain rating, and patient's level of function with gait and transfers. Variables will be discussed in greater detail in subsequent chapters.

Experimental Research Design

Experimental research investigates a cause-and-effect relationship between variables—in other words, does the independent variable x cause a change in the dependent variable y?[2-3,5,6] This category of research can be identified by several characteristics, such as random assignment to groups, a comparison group or groups, and manipulation of an independent variable. **Random assignment** means that each subject chosen for the study has an equal chance of being assigned to a specific group. Random assignment and random selection are not interchangeable terms. As we defined previously, *random selection* means that each individual in the population of interest has an equal chance of being selected for the sample. Random selection ensures that the sample is representative of the population from which it was selected. Random assignment occurs after the sample is selected and ensures that the groups are essentially the same.

The second characteristic is the use of a comparison group. A **comparison group** is a group of subjects used for comparison with an experimental group or groups. A commonly used comparison group is a control group. The control group in a study may receive no treatment, a placebo treatment, or the standard treatment while the experimental group receives the treatment under investigation.[5] A control group in a pill drug study might receive a placebo pill—if the subjects received no pill, they would obviously know they were not in the test group! A control group in a study investigating a new exercise protocol might be asked to perform the standard exercise program previously being used to compare with the new exercise protocol.

The third characteristic of an experimental design is manipulation of an independent variable. In other words, the investigator must be able to control certain aspects of the variable being studied in order to make a comparison. Examples of manipulation would be controlling the dosage of a physical agent or controlling the type or intensity of an exercise program.[2,5,7]

Experimental research is a type of quantitative research. **Quantitative research** can be defined as research that collects data in numerical form and utilizes statistical methods for analysis.[4] Studies that are typically classified as experimental designs are true experiments and quasi-experiments. The randomized controlled trial (RCT) is an example of true experimental design. Quasi-experimental design may be used in clinical research when it is not possible to randomly assign patients to groups or to include a control group. A study is considered quasi-experimental when it lacks either random assignment or a control group or both. Experimental research will be explored in more detail in Chapter 5.

Exploratory Research Design

Exploratory research investigates relationships between variables—in other words, is a change in variable x related to a change in variable y? Rather than being experimental, this type of research is considered observational because variables are not being manipulated. An investigator may choose an exploratory research design to predict the effect of one variable on another or to identify diagnostic factors. One specific type of exploratory research is called **methodological research**, which involves developing and testing a new measurement tool that can be used in the clinical setting.[2] An exploratory research design may involve data collection that is retrospective or prospective. A **retrospective** study involves the analysis of data that was collected in the past, such as data from patient medical records. An example of a retrospective study would be an investigation of medical records to identify possible variables (e.g., increased age, multiple diagnoses, compliance with physician instruction) that predict readmission to the hospital within 30 days. A **prospective** study involves data collection from a defined point of time and moving forward.[8] As an example, a prospective study might investigate the use of a new outcome measurement form by administering it to patients being seen in a therapy clinic. Exploratory research will be discussed in more detail in Chapter 6.

Descriptive Research Design

Descriptive research investigates and documents variables of the population of interest—in other words, what are the characteristics of the sample and do the characteristics change over time? As an example, a descriptive study might investigate trunk strength in individuals of different age groups 1 year after lumbar laminectomy. A specific type of descriptive research is called **normative research**, which involves describing standard values for a characteristic in a population.[2] How do you know what the normal hip extension range of motion would be for a 65-year-old individual? How can you determine if your 85-year-old patient's walking speed is normal? Normative studies are conducted to provide a basis for comparison to a normal value in the clinical setting. Another specific type of descriptive research is called **qualitative research**, which attempts to explore and describe human experiences through the individual's perspective.[9] An example of qualitative research would be a study to explore patient perceptions about the impact of the Affordable Care Act on their health and well-being. Descriptive research will be described in greater detail in Chapter 7.

SUMMARY

The purpose of this chapter was to introduce terminology that is commonly used in research. The design of a research study must be appropriate for the research question being asked. Studies may be designed to investigate cause and effect, investigate the relationship between variables, or describe the attributes of a population. A study should be valid, and the research methods should be reliable. A sample is typically chosen for a study from the accessible population of interest. A sample can be selected by using either probability or nonprobability sampling methods. Simple random sampling and cluster sampling are two examples of probability sampling. Examples of nonprobability sampling are convenience sampling and snowball sampling. One category of research is experimental, which includes true experiments and quasi-experiments. A second category of research is exploratory, which is considered observational rather than experimental. A third category is descriptive research, which includes normative and qualitative studies. Each category of research will be investigated in more detail in the following chapters.

● Case Scenario

A colleague, who knows that you have an interest in current research related to stroke, has provided you with a copy of a research report from the *Physical Therapy Journal*. The article describes walking activity of individuals with stroke compared with older adults without disability. The researchers recruited volunteers for the study from community-dwelling individuals in the local area. They invited all individuals older than 18 years who were post-stroke as well as older individuals without disability to participate in the study. Participants were recruited from local physical therapy clinics and stroke support groups as well as through newspaper advertisements for a period of 16 months. The study participants included 54 individuals who were post-stroke and 18 individuals without disability.

CASE QUESTIONS

1. What type of sample did the researchers use for this study?

_____

_____

2. What are some other methods the researchers could have used to obtain a sample for this study?

_____

_____

3. Why do you think the number of individuals without disability was so much lower than the number of individuals post-stroke?

_____

_____

4. Do you think the results of this study could be generalized to all patients who are post-stroke?

_____

_____

Review Activities

1. In your own words, explain the difference between reliability and validity.

   _____

   _____

   _____

   _____

2. Briefly explain the importance of the concept of bias in research.

   _____

   _____

   _____

   _____

3. Compare and contrast a population and a sample.

   _____

   _____

   _____

   _____

4. List and define two types of probability sampling.

   _____

   _____

   _____

   _____

5. List and define two types of nonprobability sampling.

   _____

   _____

   _____

   _____

6. Identify the purpose and two distinguishing characteristics of:
   a. Experimental research

   _____

   _____

   _____

   _____

b. Exploratory research

_____

_____

_____

_____

c. Descriptive research

_____

_____

_____

_____

MATCHING

_____ 1. Reliability   A. Variable being manipulated

_____ 2. Validity   B. Sampling method most likely to result in representative sample

_____ 3. Sample   C. Method in which every individual has an equal chance of being selected for sample

_____ 4. Generalization   D. Producing same results each time

_____ 5. Random selection   E. Variable being measured as outcome

_____ 6. Random assignment   F. Accuracy of measurement or conclusion

_____ 7. Independent variable   G. Subset of a population

_____ 8. Dependent variable   H. Ability to apply results of study to population

_____ 9. Probability sampling   I. Method in which each subject has equal chance of being in a specific group

_____ 10. Nonprobability sampling   J. Method of sampling that is not random

References

1. Field A. *Discovering Statistics Using SPSS.* 3rd ed. Thousand Oaks, CA: Sage Publications; 2009.
2. Portney LG, Watkins MP. *Foundations of Clinical Research: Applications to Practice.* Upper Saddle River, NJ: Pearson Education; 2008.
3. Hack LM, Gwyer J. *Evidence into Practice: Integrating Judgment, Values, and Research.* Philadelphia, PA: F. A. Davis; 2013.
4. Pannucci CJ, Wilkins EG. Identifying and avoiding bias in research. *Plast Reconstr Surg.* 2010;126(2):619-625.

5. Research Methods Knowledge Base. http://www.socialresearchmethods.net. Accessed July 2, 2015.

6. Pyrczak F. *Evaluating Research in Academic Journals: A Practical Guide to Realistic Evaluation.* 4th ed. Glendale, CA: Fred Pyrczak; 2008.

7. Mertler CA, Vannatta RA. *Advanced and Multivariate Statistical Methods: Practical Application and Interpretation.* 4th ed. Glendale, CA: Fred Pyrczak; 2010.

8. Helewa A, Walker JM. *Critical Evaluation of Research in Physical Rehabilitation.* Philadelphia, PA: W. B. Saunders; 2000.

9. Fetters L, Tilson J. *Evidence Based Physical Therapy.* Philadelphia, PA: F. A. Davis; 2012.

Experimental Research

Chapter at a Glance

Learning Outcomes

After reading this chapter, the reader will be able to:

· Differentiate between true experiments and quasi-experiments.
· Describe the key components that define a randomized controlled trial (RCT).
· Describe common research designs for true experiments and quasi-experiments.
· Explain key differences between an independent groups design and a repeated measures design.
· Identify common threats and biases that may challenge the validity of a study.

Key Terms

· Active (positive) control group
· Between-subjects design
· Blinding
· Carryover effect
· Control group
· Crossover design
· Double-blind study
· Experimental group
· Factorial design
· Independent groups design
· Nonparametric tests
· No-treatment control group
· One-way (single-factor) design
· Parametric tests
· Placebo control group
· Post-test
· Pre-test
· Quasi-experimental design
· Repeated measures design
· Single-blind study
· Washout period
· Within-subjects design

◘ FOOD FOR THOUGHT

You are a physical therapist assistant working in a large inpatient rehabilitation hospital. Your facility has recently begun accepting more patients with traumatic brain injury. Although you have some experience with treating this diagnosis, you would like to review some research articles to improve your knowledge about specific interventions for patients at different levels of cognitive functioning (e.g., Rancho Los Amigos scale). During your literature search, you find a report on a study that investigated the use of a virtual game system compared with standard balance training for patients after a traumatic brain injury. The study was conducted in a rehabilitation hospital and included 100 subjects (50 in each group). The authors reported that, although there was no significant difference in balance scores between the groups, the virtual game system group demonstrated a higher level of satisfaction with therapy and a higher rate of compliance with scheduled therapy treatment time. The study is identified as a randomized controlled trial.

Questions to consider:

· Would this article be helpful to you? Why or why not?
· Does the number of subjects seem reasonable?
· Do the results seem to support the use of a virtual game system?

Introduction

This chapter will provide an explanation of experimental research and examples of a variety of experimental research designs. The purpose of this chapter is to prepare the reader to critically appraise experimental research articles during a literature search. Experimental research investigates a cause-and-effect relationship between variables, and the research question will ask: Does the independent variable x cause a change in the dependent variable y? This type of research is primarily used for intervention studies, such as looking at the effects of a particular physical agent, exercise, or mobilization technique on patient outcomes. Articles that reflect different types of research designs will be presented to assist the reader in understanding this topic.

Experimental research is considered the most rigorous type of research, with the randomized controlled trial (RCT) often cited as the gold standard of research design for intervention studies.[1] Experimental research includes RCTs and quasi-experiments and investigates the effect of one or more independent variables on one or more dependent variables. To provide clarity for comparison of the different types of research designs, examples in this chapter will use reports of studies investigating interventions on low back pain.

Experimental Research Design

Experimental research design primarily includes two categories: true experiments, or RCTs, and quasi-experiments.[1] An RCT is a study in which subjects are assigned randomly to groups to receive one of several interventions, of which one intervention may be a control group. An RCT must include more than one group for comparison, and subjects must be randomly assigned to groups. If a study does not meet these criteria, it is considered to be quasi-experimental. A **quasi-experimental design** means that either (1) subjects were not randomly assigned to groups or (2) a comparison group was not used.[1-3]

One component of research design is the timing of the test or measurement that will be used to compare groups. A **pre-test** is a test or measurement administered before the experiment or intervention. The use of a pre-test allows the researcher to compare groups to determine whether the groups are similar before the intervention. It would also allow a researcher to use the change in a subject's status as a dependent variable. A **post-test** is a test or measurement administered after the experiment or intervention. Experimental designs commonly use both a pre-test and a post-test.[2-4] However, you may find a study that included only a post-test for a particular reason. For example, a study comparing two different types of anesthesia on an individual's functional level on postoperative day 1 following hip fracture repair would not include a pre-test because a hip fracture is an unexpected event.

Another design feature is the number of factors, or independent variables, involved as well as the number of levels of each factor. Recall from Chapter 4 that the independent variable is the one being manipulated by the researcher. A research design may include only one factor, such as an exercise program or ultrasound intervention. This type of design is called a **one-way,** or **single-factor**, **design.**[1-4] In a study that is comparing a new exercise program with a standard exercise program, the independent variable would have two levels: (1) exercise intervention A, or new exercise program; and (2) exercise intervention B, or standard exercise program. A single-factor design can have any number of levels, and the researcher will determine the number of levels based on a variety of factors (i.e., research question, cost, time, availability of subjects). A more complicated research design would be a **factorial design,** which would include two or more independent variables, or factors. Factorial design may be further classified by the number of factors included in the study, such as a two-way (two factors) or three-way (three factors) design.[2-4] An example of a two-way design would be a study in which investigators wanted to compare a new exercise program to a standard exercise program but also wanted to determine whether it would make a difference if the subjects completed the exercise program twice a day compared with every other day (frequency). Using this design, the investigators would need to assign subjects to four groups: experimental group performing exercises twice a day, experimental group performing exercises every other day, standard group performing exercises twice a day, and standard exercise group performing exercises every other day. Table 5.1 diagrams the two-way design.

Randomized Controlled Trials

Let's review the key factors that define an RCT (Box 5-1). One key factor is the identification of independent variables that can be manipulated by the investigator. Another factor is random assignment of subjects to groups. Random assignment will increase the likelihood that groups will be similar at the beginning of the study. Additionally, an RCT must include at least two groups for comparison. Although the investigator

Table 5.1 | Two-Way Research Design

		Frequency	
		Once per Day	**Every Other Day**
Exercise	Experimental exercise program	Group E1	Group E2
	Standard exercise program	Group S1	Group S2

Box 5.1 | Three Key Characteristics of a Randomized Controlled Trial

- Independent variable(s) that can be manipulated
- Random assignment of subjects to groups
- At least two groups for comparisons

---

may decide to include a control group as one of the groups, a control group is not required. And finally, the investigator should minimize threats that might affect the outcome of the study. Blinding or masking is an important factor in minimizing potential bias. **Blinding,** also called masking, is defined as a method for ensuring that individuals involved in a study do not know the group assignment of the subjects.[4] A **single-blind study** would be a study in which one of the parties involved (researcher, subject) was blinded but not the other. A **double-blind study** means that neither the subjects nor the researcher are aware of the group assignment during the study.

The design of an RCT is commonly categorized as either an independent groups design or repeated measures design. **Independent groups design** means that subjects are assigned to and participate in only one group (i.e., experimental group or control group but not both). This design is also referred to as **between-subjects design** because comparisons are made between subjects in one group and subjects in another group. Independent groups design requires a larger number of subjects but may be completed in less time because subjects are only completing one condition of the experiment. **Repeated measures design** means that each subject participates in each condition of the experiment—in other words, both the experimental group or groups and the control group—over a period of time. This design is also referred to as **within-subjects design** because comparisons are made between a single subject's performance in one condition (i.e., experimental group) and the same subject's performance in another condition (i.e., control group). Each subject in repeated measures designs acts as his or her own control. This design can be completed with fewer subjects but requires more time because subjects are completing all conditions of the experiment.[1-4]

Independent Groups Design

When two independent groups are used, the two groups commonly included are an experimental group and a control group (Fig. 5.1 and Table 5.2). The **experimental group** is the group of subjects who will undergo the experimental intervention. The **control group** is the group of subjects who will not receive the experimental intervention and are used as a comparison for the experimental group. The control group may receive no treatment, a placebo treatment, or the standard treatment.[2] When the control group receives the standard treatment, the investigators often refer to the group as an intervention group. You may also see these groups referred to as follows:

- **No-treatment control group,** when the subjects in the control group receive no treatment
- **Placebo control group,** when the subjects in the control group receive a placebo treatment
- **Active (positive) control group,** when the subjects receive the standard treatment

The investigators will determine the type of control group to use based on scientific and ethical principles. The active control group design is commonly used when it is not reasonable or ethical to use a placebo treatment. For example, it could be considered unethical to provide no treatment to subjects with a serious condition when a standard treatment is known to be effective. Investigators in that instance could decide to use the standard treatment as the active control. An independent groups design could

Independent Group Design

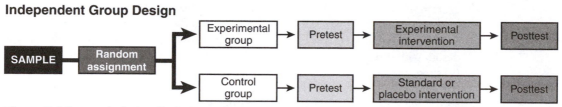

Figure 5.1 Research design for independent groups.

include two experimental or intervention groups and no control group. In that instance, the groups are compared with each other rather than a control. By definition, an RCT must include a comparison group (two groups to compare) but does not require that one of the groups is a control group. An RCT may also include more than two groups, for example, two experimental groups and a control group, or three intervention groups. Keep in mind, however, that the more independent groups an experiment uses, the greater the number of subjects needed for the study. Let's take a look at some examples of independent groups designs.

A report in the *Journal of Physical Therapy* from March 2005 was titled, "Trunk Muscle Stabilization Training Plus General Exercise Versus General Exercise Only: Randomized Controlled Trial of Patients With Recurrent Low Back Pain."[6] Subjects included 55 participants who were randomly assigned to either a stabilization-enhanced exercise group ($n = 29$) or a general exercise-only group ($n = 26$). Subjects completed outcome questionnaires before and after the intervention as well as 3 months after the end of the intervention period. This study was an RCT using an independent groups design and would be classified as a single-factor design with two levels. The factor would be exercise with levels of (1) stabilization-enhanced or (2) general exercise. The study incorporated a pre-test before the intervention and two post-tests after the intervention. It was a double-blind study because both the subjects and the investigators were blinded to group assignment. The authors reported that the two groups were both intervention groups; however, the general exercise (only group could also have been called an active control group. The study found that both groups demonstrated improved outcomes, and the only significant difference between groups was with self-reported disability. The general exercise group demonstrated more improvement immediately after the intervention period, but no difference was found between groups after 3 months.

A second article from the *Journal of Physical Therapy* in October 2010 was titled, "Motor Control Exercises, Sling Exercises, and General Exercises for Patients With Chronic Low Back Pain: A Randomized Controlled Trial With 1-Year Follow-up."[7] Subjects included 109 participants who were randomly assigned to one of three groups: low-load motor control exercises ($n = 36$), high-load sling exercises ($n = 36$), or general

Table 5.2 | Examples of Independent Groups Design Configurations

Experimental intervention	+	No-treatment Control
Experimental Intervention	+	Placebo (sham) Control
Experimental Intervention	+	Active (standard treatment) Control
Experimental intervention A	+	Experimental Intervention B

exercises ($n = 37$). Subjects completed outcome questionnaires before and after the intervention as well as 1 year after the end of the intervention period. This study was an RCT using an independent groups design and would be classified as a single-factor design with three levels. The factor would be exercise with levels of (1) motor control, (2) sling, and (3) general. The study incorporated a pre-test before the intervention and two post-tests after the intervention. The study was single-blinded because the investigators were blinded to group assignment but the subjects were not. The authors reported that all three groups were intervention groups; however, the general exercise group could also have been called an active control group. The results showed no significant differences between the three groups on outcome measures.

Repeated Measures Design

In repeated measures design, every subject participates in each condition of the experiment. This design controls for individual differences among subjects because all subjects complete all activities. However, this design also includes the potential for carryover effects. **Carryover effect** can be defined as the effect of one intervention continuing into the next test period. As an example of repeated measures, consider a design that included an intervention group and a control group with a testing period of 4 weeks. All subjects for the study would complete a pre-test, then complete the control group activity (if any) for 4 weeks followed by another test. Next, all subjects would complete the intervention group activity for 4 weeks, followed by the post-test. If necessary, a period of time called the washout period would occur between the first test period and the second test period. A **washout period** is a period of rest between test periods that should provide time for any carryover effects of the first treatment to be eliminated.[1] With a repeated measures design, the subject's performance on the post-test is compared with the same subject's performance on the pre-test and on any intermediate tests. Figure 5.2 depicts the repeated measures design (including a washout period).

A special type of repeated measures design is the crossover design. The **crossover design** consists of a design in which groups complete the conditions of the study in a different order.[1-3] The crossover design is the most common type of repeated measures design because the effects of activity sequencing are taken into account (Fig. 5.3). In a crossover study, the subjects are randomly assigned to groups, and the groups then complete the conditions of the study in different sequences. For example, the study could be set up as follows: one group of subjects would complete the control group activity for 4 weeks, followed by the washout period, then the intervention group activity for 4 weeks. The other group of subjects would complete the activities in reverse order: intervention group activity for 4 weeks, followed by the washout period, then the control group activity for 4 weeks. Let's take a look at an example of a repeated measures study.

Repeated Measures Design

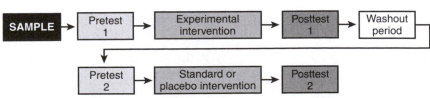

Figure 5.2 Research design for repeated measures.

Repeated Measures Crossover Design

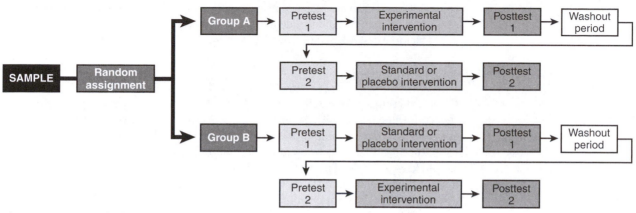

Figure 5.3 Research design for repeated measures crossover design.

An article published in the March/April 2007 study of the *Journal of Manipulative and Physiological Therapeutics* was titled, "Flexion Mobilizations With Movement Techniques: The Immediate Effects on Range of Movement and Pain in Subjects With Low Back Pain."[8] The study included 26 subjects with low back pain and pain on lumbar flexion. The subjects received two interventions in random order during one therapy session: One intervention consisted of flexion mobilizations with movement techniques (MWMs), and the other intervention was a placebo. Subjects were tested for spinal range of motion and pain rating before interventions, after the first intervention, and after the second intervention. This study was an RCT using a repeated measures design and would be classified as a single-factor design with two levels: (1) mobilization and (2) no mobilization (placebo). The study incorporated a pre-test before the intervention and a post-test after each intervention. It was a single-blind study because the investigator conducting the measurements was blinded to intervention order. The results indicated that the MWM group significantly increased range of motion immediately following intervention compared with the control group, but no other differences were identified.

In summary, RCTs can use either an independent groups design or a repeated measures design. Independent groups design is called between-subjects design because comparisons are made between groups. Repeated measures design is called within subjects design because comparisons are made between a subject's pre-test score and the same subject's post-test score. One type of repeated measures design is the crossover design, in which groups complete the conditions of the study in different orders. RCTs typically

Learning Task

Using PubMed, locate an RCT article published during the past 5 years. Read the article and answer the following questions:

• Is the study design an independent groups design or a repeated measures design?
• Were the subjects randomly assigned to groups?
• Did the study use a pre-test, a post-test, or both?
• Was the study blinded? If so, was it a single-blind or double-blind study?
• Did the study use a control group?
• How many factors were included? How many levels?

include tests that are administered before and after the intervention period (pre-test and post-test), but in some instances the test is only administered after the intervention period (post-test). RCTs can investigate one independent variable (one-way or single-factor design) or more than one independent variable (two-way or three-way design, sometimes called factorial design). The independent variable may have two or more levels.

Quasi-Experiments

Quasi-experimental research designs often look very similar to true experimental designs but will differ in at least one key aspect. Quasi-experimental studies lack random assignment, comparison groups, or both. This research design is not as rigorous as a true experiment but may be a reasonable alternative in the clinical setting. Clinicians should keep a couple of points in mind when reviewing a quasi-experiment. If a study does not include random assignment, it is less likely that the groups will be similar or equal. If a study does not include a comparison group, it is impossible to make a comparison between an experimental intervention and a standard intervention or no intervention. In other words, subjects in the study who received an intervention may have shown improvement, but it is not possible to clearly determine whether the improvement was caused by the intervention or some other factor.

Investigators may decide to use a quasi-experimental design when random assignment is not possible because of constraints within the clinical setting. As an example, a report of a quasi-experimental study, "Comparison of Graded Exercise and Graded Exposure Clinical Outcomes for Patients With Chronic Low Back Pain," was published in the *Journal of Orthopaedic and Sports Physical Therapy* in November 2010.[9] Subjects included 33 patients enrolled in a chronic pain rehabilitation program, with 15 in the graded exercise group and 18 in the graded exposure group. The graded exercise group increased exercise and activity based on patient tolerance. The graded exposure group increased exercise and activity based on patient's level of fear of an exercise or activity (because of past experience of exercise or activity causing pain). The authors reported that they were not able to randomly assign patients to groups in this study because patients were participating in group exercise programs within the facility. They decided to use graded exercise for patients who entered the rehabilitation program during the first 8 months of the study and graded exposure during the last 8 months of the study. This study was a quasi-experimental study using an independent groups design and would be classified as a single-factor design with two levels. The factor would be treatment with levels of (1) graded exercise and (2) graded exposure. The study incorporated a pre-test before the intervention and a post-test after the intervention. The study was not blinded because of clinical limitations. The authors reported that both groups were intervention groups, so no control group was included. Both groups showed improvements in pain and disability levels, and no differences were found between the two groups.

Learning Task
Using the CINAHL search engine, locate an article about a quasi-experimental study published within the past 10 years. Read the article and answer the following questions:
• Were the subjects randomly assigned to groups?
• Was there a comparison group?
• Was the study blinded? If so, was it a single-blind or double-blind study?
• Did the study include a pre-test, a post-test, or both?
• How many factors were included? How many levels?

Putting It All Together

To assist the reader with understanding some of the components of experimental research design, let's look at an example of an experimental clinical study.

Joanna is a physical therapist assistant (PTA) in a busy orthopedic outpatient clinic, and she works as part of a team with Brian, a physical therapist (PT). Brian and Joanna have developed a core stabilization program for patients presenting with low back pain. They believe that their patients have better outcomes for function and core strength than those who perform the standard exercise program that has been used by the clinic for several years. Brian and Joanna would like to conduct a small study to determine whether there is actually a difference in outcomes between interventions, with a time frame of 6 weeks for performing the exercises.

- Brian and Joanna decide to conduct a pre-test and a post-test in order to be able to investigate the change in function and core stability for subjects. The subjects will be tested and measured for function and for core strength initially and then will be tested and measured again after the 6-week exercise period.
- Brian and Joanna decide to use three groups:
  - The first group will perform the new exercise program as well as receive education in proper body mechanics (experimental intervention group A).
  - The second group will perform the standard exercise program as well as receive education in proper body mechanics (standard intervention group B).
  - The final group will only receive education in proper body mechanics (control group).
  This would be considered a one-way design, with one factor (exercise program) and three levels (experimental, standard, and control). Brian and Joanna could have decided to use two groups, with one group performing the new exercise program and the second group performing the standard exercise program. The two-group design would still be considered a one-way design, with one factor and two levels.
- Brian and Joanna choose to use an independent groups design. They will plan to recruit 45 subjects in order to assign 15 subjects to each of the three groups. As subjects are enrolled, they will be randomly assigned to one of the three groups. Each subject will only participate in one group. The investigators could have set up their study as a repeated measures crossover design by randomly assigning subjects to either Group A or Group B. Group A could complete the new exercise program, followed by a washout period, then the general exercise program. Group B could complete the general exercise program, followed by a washout period, then the new exercise program.
- Brian and Joanna could have set up their study as quasi-experimental by:
  - Allowing subjects to select the group in which they preferred to participate (lack of random assignment)
  - Assigning all subjects to one group, with that group completing the new core stabilization program (lack of comparison group).

Addressing Biases and Threats

The information provided in this chapter regarding experimental research should be helpful to the reader in reviewing and understanding this type of evidence. The true experiment, or RCT, is often considered the gold standard for interventional studies. Quasi-experimental studies can also provide useful information for clinicians as long as the reader understands the potential biases involved in this type of design. Investigators can take specific steps to control factors that might introduce bias or threats to validity. We have already discussed a couple of important considerations. The use of a control group can help the researcher and the reader decide that any change is due to the independent variable, as long as the groups are equal at the beginning of the study. Random assignment is a mechanism for trying to ensure that the groups are as equal as possible. Let's review other key components of addressing threats and biases in experimental research.

Blinding

Blinding or masking is a mechanism that should minimize bias. Think about our scenario at the ABC Clinic. Brian and Joanna have developed a new exercise program that they believe provides better outcomes than the standard program. This belief could affect their objectivity in measuring outcomes if they are aware of a subject's grouping. If possible, they could ensure that the individual measuring the subjects' outcomes is not informed about each subject's grouping. Studies may also be set up to include blinding of the patient because a patient's perception could influence his or her performance. In some scenarios, blinding or masking is difficult if not impossible.

Tests and Measures

Another threat to the validity of a study revolves around obtaining outcome measures. If the outcome measure is a questionnaire, for example, post-test responses may improve because the subject is familiar with the questions from the pre-test. The subjects may also become more aware of expected responses during the intervention period. The skill of the investigator with a measuring instrument or the sensitivity of the measuring instrument can also affect the results. The study should use outcome measures and tools that show good reliability in the method for which they are being used (i.e., test-retest reliability, interrater reliability). Reliability is defined as the consistency of a measurement tool. The measurement tool should also demonstrate good validity, which is defined as the accuracy of a tool (i.e., face validity, concurrent validity).

Sample Size

Small sample size can be another threat to a study's results. With a small number of subjects, it is more difficult to ensure that the groups will be equivalent, and it is more likely that a single subject's differences will affect the results. A study may begin with a reasonable number of subjects, but losing subjects because of attrition (i.e., illness, dropout, noncompliance) can result in too small a number completing the study. Investigators have to take attrition into account when they determine the sample size needed for the study. They also must balance the need for a large number of subjects with the reality of time and costs involved with recruiting and studying larger groups. An investigator may have difficulty finding enough available subjects when a study is investigating an unusual condition or diagnosis.

Groups

For studies that use more than one group, the treatments should be as equivalent as possible, and extraneous activities and interventions should be minimized. In our scenario for ABC clinic, Brian and Joanna decided to use three groups for their study. Two groups would be performing exercises and receiving instruction in body mechanics, and the third group would only receive instruction in body mechanics. To keep the treatments as equivalent as possible, the investigators should ensure that the time spent at the clinic as well as the frequency of visits was equal across all three groups. Participants should be informed not to start any other new activity or intervention during the study period because this could affect the validity of the study. Do you think it might affect the outcome of Brian and Joanna's study if several participants in the experimental group decided to meet on their own at a local gym for a core-strengthening class twice a week during the study? Because one of the dependent variables was core strength, the local gym activity would likely affect the results. Investigators should find out about other activities, treatments, and medications for all of the subjects and ensure that these do not change during the study.

Statistical Testing

Another key consideration is the use of appropriate statistical tests when analyzing the data collected during a study. A study may have a sound research design, but if the investigator uses the wrong statistical procedure to analyze the results, the conclusions may not be valid. As an example, a number of statistical tests are categorized as either parametric or nonparametric. **Parametric** tests make a number of assumptions about the population distribution and the data being collected. If the data collected during a study do not meet the assumptions of the test being used, a nonparametric test should be used. **Nonparametric** tests do not generally make assumptions about the populations or the data being collected.

The authors of research articles should include a discussion of the limitations of the study, and the clinician should read this discussion to be more informed. In many instances, the limitations discussed by the authors are potential threats to the validity of the results. The authors might note that their sample size was small and explain their rationale for choosing the sample size. The authors might identify the limitations of the selected placebo treatment and explain their rationale for using that particular placebo treatment. For studies that were not blinded, the authors typically will provide an explanation about why blinding was not possible. Authors should also provide some discussion about whether the results of the study can be generalized to a larger population. In the end, the clinician reading the article is responsible for determining whether the authors' discussion and conclusions are reasonable. The clinician can then decide whether the results are applicable to the clinical question or patient situation.

Application to Evidence Based Practice

Is it important for a clinician to be able to read and understand an experimental research article? Should a clinician be able to appraise the quality of an RCT report? The answer to both questions is yes. Most resources on evidence based practice recommend that clinicians focus a search for evidence on systematic reviews or meta-analyses and clinical practice guidelines. However, a clinician could easily have a clinical question that has not been addressed in a systematic review or clinical guideline. If the clinician is able to locate an RCT or a quasi-experimental article, the clinician must be able to appraise the article to determine whether it should be used. A clinician should be able to identify the type of experimental research as well as the type of research design. The clinician should also be able to determine whether the research design seems to be appropriate for answering the research question. Both the PT and the PTA, as part of a PT/PTA team, should be able to determine the quality of evidence provided by experimental research articles. They should be able to identify potential sources of bias and threats and determine whether the investigators addressed them adequately. Experimental research is primarily used to investigate interventions, which is the primary component of physical therapy practice that involves the PTA. Experimental research plays an important role in expanding the knowledge base in physical therapy and provides a resource for the PT or PTA involved in evidence based practice.

SUMMARY

This chapter has covered types of experimental research and various research designs that are commonly encountered during a clinician's search for evidence. The two primary categories of experimental research are randomized controlled trials and quasi-experimental studies. A study can be designed to include a pre-test, a post-test, or both and can be categorized based on the number of independent variables being investigated. RCTs can be designed using independent groups or repeated measures and must include a comparison group, such as a control group. RCTs also must include random assignment of subjects to groups. Quasi-experimental studies lack random assignment, comparison groups, or both. Experimental research investigates a cause-and-effect relationship between variables and is considered the most rigorous type of research for interventional studies. PTs and PTAs should be able to read, understand, and appraise an experimental research article as part of a PT/PTA team utilizing evidence in practice.

● Case Scenario

You are a PTA working in a large academic research hospital. During lunch, you overhear one of the therapists describing a research study that she is designing with a team of therapists and neurologists. The study will investigate whether earlier mobilization of a patient following cerebrovascular accident (within 24 hours of hospital admission) would result in better functional outcomes than not mobilizing the patient until 24 to 48 hours after hospital admission (current practice). The therapy treatment will be the same for both groups; the only difference will be the time frame after admission. Patients will be assigned to the early mobilization group or the standard mobilization group using a computer program for randomization. Outcome measures will be taken before discharge from the hospital and again when the patient returns to the neurologist's office for a 1-month follow-up visit. The therapists and neurologists will have access to information about the patient's group assignment.

CASE QUESTIONS

1. How would you classify the type of study?

_____

_____

2. What is the group design?

_____

_____

3. Were subjects randomized to groups appropriately?

_____

_____

4. Was blinding/masking included in the study?

_____

_____

5. Can you think of a change to the research design that might have improved the study?

_____

_____

Review Activities

1. In your own words, explain the difference between a randomized controlled trial and a quasi-experiment.

   _____

   _____

   _____

   _____

2. List three key factors that define a randomized controlled trial.

   _____

   _____

   _____

   _____

3. Briefly explain the difference between independent groups design and repeated measures designs.

   _____

   _____

   _____

   _____

4. List and define three types of control groups.

   _____

   _____

   _____

   _____

5. Provide an example of a one-way design.

   _____

   _____

   _____

   _____

6. List three examples of threats to the validity of a study.

   _____

   _____

   _____

   _____

MATCHING

_____ 1. One-way design   A. Each subject participates in each condition

_____ 2. Factorial design   B. Effect of one intervention continuing into next test period

_____ 3. Independent groups design   C. Another name for repeated measures design

_____ 4. Between-subjects design   D. Control group receives a sham intervention

_____ 5. Within-subjects design   E. Period of rest

_____ 6. Active control group   F. Subjects participate in only one group

_____ 7. Placebo control group   G. Study includes one independent variable

_____ 8. Carryover effect   H. Control group receives standard treatment

_____ 9. Washout period   I. Study includes two or more variables

_____ 10. Repeated measures design   J. Another name for independent groups design

▬ References

1. Portney LG, Watkins MP. *Foundations of Clinical Research: Applications to Practice.* Upper Saddle River, NJ: Pearson Education; 2008.
2. Research Methods Knowledge Base. http://www.socialresearchmethods.net/kb/index.php. Accessed July 6, 2015.
3. Fetters L, Tilson J. *Evidence Based Physical Therapy.* Philadelphia, PA: F. A. Davis; 2012.
4. Field A. *Discovering Statistics Using SPSS.* 3rd ed. Thousand Oaks, CA: Sage Publications; 2009.
5. Mertler CA, Vannatta RA. *Advanced and Multivariate Statistical Methods: Practical Application and Interpretation.* 4th ed. Glendale, CA: Fred Pyrczak; 2010.
6. Koumantakis GA, Watson PJ, Oldham JA. Trunk muscle stabilization training plus general exercise versus general exercise only: randomized controlled trial of patients with recurrent low back pain. *Phys Ther.* 2005;85(3):209-225.
7. Unsgaard-Tondel M, Fladmark AM, Salvesen O, Vasseljen O. Motor control exercises, sling exercises, and general exercises for patients with chronic low back pain: a randomized controlled trial with 1-year follow-up. *Phys Ther.* 2010;90(10):1426-1440.
8. Konstantinou K, Foster N, Rushton A, Baxter D, Wright C, Breen A. Flexion mobilizations with movement techniques: the immediate effects on range of movement and pain in subjects with low back pain. *J Manipulative Physiol Ther.* 2007;30(3):178-185.
9. George SZ, Wittmer VT, Fillingim RB, Robinson ME. Comparison of graded exercise and graded exposure clinical outcomes for patients with chronic low back pain. *J Orthop Sports Phys Ther.* 2010;40(11):694-704.

Exploratory Research

Chapter at a Glance

Learning Outcomes

After reading this chapter, the reader will be able to:

· Discuss the various types of exploratory research.
· Describe similarities and differences between a cohort study and a case-control study.
· Describe similarities and differences between a longitudinal study and a cross-sectional study.
· Compare and contrast the characteristics of retrospective and prospective studies.
· Identify the role of methodological research in physical therapy practice.
· Discuss the application of exploratory research to evidence based practice.

Key Terms

· Case-control study
· Cases
· Clinical decision rule
· Cohort
· Cohort study
· Controls
· Correlational study
· Cross-sectional study
· Longitudinal study
· Predictive study
· Prospective study
· Retrospective study

◘ FOOD FOR THOUGHT

Leslie is a relatively new physical therapist assistant working in a pediatric outpatient clinic. Melissa, a physical therapist, evaluated a patient this morning and asked Leslie to assist with this patient during the next few visits. The 6-year-old patient's diagnosis is cerebral palsy with spastic quadriplegia. Leslie has not worked with any patients with quadriplegic spasticity, so she decided to review the literature before the patient returned for the next visit. She located a recent report that examined the relationship between spasticity, weakness, balance, gross motor function, and activity limitation in children with cerebral palsy. The study included 61 children with cerebral palsy who had either spastic diplegia or spastic hemiplegia. The authors identified the study as a longitudinal cohort study, which means the authors followed a group of children over a period of time.

Questions to consider:
· Would this article be helpful to Leslie? Why or why not?
· Does the number of subjects seem reasonable?
· Do you think the authors could have gotten the same type of information by looking at a large group of children at one point in time (i.e., age 4 or age 6 years)?

Introduction

This chapter will provide an explanation of exploratory research and examples of various types of research categorized as exploratory. The purpose of this chapter is to prepare the reader to critically appraise exploratory research articles during a literature search, so examples of exploratory research articles will be presented to allow practice in reviewing and appraising. Exploratory research is defined as research that investigates data to determine the relationship between variables.[1-3] The research question will ask: Is a change in variable x *related to* a change in variable y? This is in contrast to experimental research, which investigates a cause and effect (does the variable *x cause* a change in variable *y*?). Exploratory research can identify a relationship between variables but does not explain cause and effect. For example, in 2011 Barron and Guidon investigated the relationship between grip strength and balance to determine whether grip strength might be used as a screening tool for impaired balance.[4] The investigators hypothesized that decreased grip strength and impaired balance would have some of the same underlying factors in older people and therefore might decline at the same time (i.e., be related). Clearly, they were not attempting to demonstrate that decreased grip strength might cause impaired balance or increased risk for falling.

Exploratory research includes a wide range of research designs, including cohort studies, case-control studies, correlation and prediction, and methodological research. Exploratory studies can be classified as either longitudinal or cross-sectional. A **longitudinal study** follows a group of subjects over time and collects data at repeated intervals.[1,3] A group of subjects followed over time is called a **cohort** and may be grouped together based on a variety of factors, such as location, age, or event. For example, an investigator might choose to follow residents who lived near the nuclear power plant in Japan damaged by a tsunami in 2011, with the purpose of identifying health issues that arise over a period of years. A **cross-sectional study** investigates groups of subjects at one point in time and compares the characteristics of the different groups.[1,3] In this type of study, the groups may be categorized based on a characteristic such as age, gender, or country of birth. An example would be an investigation of current opinions of health-care reform across different age groups. Figure 6.1 provides a comparison of longitudinal and cross-sectional studies.

Exploratory research can also be classified as either retrospective or prospective. A **retrospective study** is an investigation of data that have already been collected in the past. These data can be collected from existing databases or existing medical records. Retrospective studies frequently use data from medical records. A **prospective study** collects new data during a specified period of time. The investigator will plan for the collection of data and can ensure that data collection procedures are followed appropriately. Retrospective studies are typically less expensive and less time-consuming than prospective studies, but there are also disadvantages. The investigator does not have any control over the collection of the data in a retrospective study because the data have already been collected. When data are collected from medical records, for example, each record may not include all of the data points being investigated, so the records that lack the data cannot be used. Tests or measures may not have been conducted on each patient, or the test might not have been recorded in such a way that the information is identifiable. There is also no way to determine whether individuals collecting the data were administering the tests correctly or reliably. A prospective study, because it is a planned collection of data, can ensure that participants will have all of the tests or measures conducted. Depending on the circumstances, prospective studies are typically preferable to retrospective studies. Figure 6.2 provides a comparison of retrospective and prospective studies.

Exploratory research as a whole investigates the relationship between two or more variables and may attempt to determine whether a change in one variable can predict a change in another variable. To provide clarity for comparison of the different types of research designs, examples in this chapter will use reports of studies investigating balance or falls.

Cohort Studies

One type of exploratory research is the cohort study. A **cohort study** is a study that follows a specific cohort, or group, over a period of time.[1] Participants enter the study before they have acquired the condition of interest in order to identify factors that contribute to the development of the condition. Because this type of study follows a group or groups over time, it is considered a longitudinal study. Cohort studies can be conducted for a variety of reasons, such as the development of a diagnostic test or measure, to determine the incidence or history of a condition, or to compare variables across categories. Cohort studies can be either prospective or retrospective, depending on the

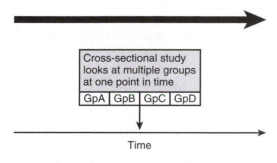

Longitudinal study follows a single group (cohort) over time with multiple measurements at specified intervals

Cross-sectional study looks at multiple groups at one point in time

GpA | GpB | GpC | GpD

Time

Figure 6.1 Longitudinal studies follow a single cohort over time, whereas cross-sectional studies look at multiple groups at one point in time.

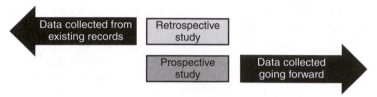

Figure 6.2 Studies utilizing retrospective designs collect data from records that already exist, whereas prospective studies collect data moving forward from the start of the study.

investigator's determination of the most appropriate research design. Because a cohort study is an exploratory study, the investigators are simply collecting observational data rather than manipulating variables or providing an intervention. Let's look at some examples.

The first study is an example of a prospective cohort study. Morrison and colleagues (2011) investigated fall rates and risk factors in elderly patients across three different health-care settings.[5] The study included 1,682 participants who were receiving physical therapy in a variety of facilities during a 1-year period. Participants were followed as long as they were receiving therapy, and any falls that occurred during their rehabilitation period were documented. The researchers developed a plan for collecting data that would ensure they had data on all of the factors they were investigating. Risk factors that were documented included participants' age, gender, diagnoses, preadmission status, previous falls, and balance. The study results revealed that individuals in an inpatient rehabilitation setting had significantly higher fall rates than individuals in other settings. Balance was a risk factor for outpatient settings but not for inpatient settings. Cognitive factors and previous history of falls were risk factors in all settings.

As a contrast to the previously described study, a retrospective study investigating the same topic would utilize data that has already been collected. Teasell and colleagues (2002) conducted a retrospective cohort study to investigate the incidence of falls on a rehabilitation unit and identify risk factors in patients after a stroke.[6] The investigators reviewed medical records for 238 consecutive patients with stroke diagnoses who had previously been admitted to the rehabilitation unit during the previous 5 years. They identified 88 patients who had fallen, with almost half of those experiencing at least two falls. The researchers found that patients who had fallen had lower scores on admission motor function assessments and were more likely to have cognitive deficits. The authors discussed a limitation of the study as its reliance on chart review, noting that only falls that were witnessed, reported, and documented were included. Patients were not necessarily asked if they had experienced a fall during their rehabilitation stay.

Learning Task
Using any search engine available, locate a cohort study article published during the past 5 years. Read the article and answer the following questions:
- Was the study prospective or retrospective?
- What were the characteristics of the cohort being studied?
- How long was the cohort followed?
- What was the research question?
- What were the results of the study?

Case-Control Studies

Another type of exploratory research is the case-control study. A **case-control study** is a study in which subjects are selected based on whether or not they have the condition being investigated.[1-3] The subjects who have the condition are called **cases**, and the subjects who do not have the condition are called **controls.** Case-control studies can be conducted for many of the same reasons as cohort studies, including development of a diagnostic test or measure or to determine the incidence or history of a condition. After the groups have been selected, the investigator will review the subjects' histories to identify risk factors for the condition, and a risk estimate can be calculated. Cases are often selected from patients in a medical setting. Controls can be selected from a variety of settings or from the population in general but should be matched to the cases on relevant factors such as age or gender. In case-control studies, it is critical that the condition being investigated is clearly defined to ensure that cases and controls are distinct from each other (Table 6.1).

The first example is a case-control study that used chronic ankle instability as the condition of interest. Linens and associates (2014) conducted a prospective study to identify postural stability tests that would identify individuals with chronic ankle instability.[7] The study included 17 cases with the condition of chronic ankle instability and 17 healthy age-matched controls. All subjects performed a number of balance tests, and the investigators determined that there were significant differences between the cases and controls on most of the tests. The investigators were then able to identify cut-off scores for the balance tests that would identify individuals with chronic ankle instability who would likely benefit from therapy to improve postural stability.

The second example of a case-control study used chronic low back pain as the condition of interest. Champagne and associates (2012) conducted a study to investigate balance and fear-avoidance factors in older women with chronic low back pain.[8] The investigators selected 15 older women with chronic low back pain and 15 age-matched pain-free controls. All subjects completed a balance confidence scale that measured confidence in performing various ambulatory activities, pain survey, and a functional mobility questionnaire. The investigators then measured a number of sensorimotor

Learning Task

Using any search engine available, locate a case-control study article published during the past 5 years. Read the article and answer the following questions:

- Was the study prospective or retrospective?
- What characteristic(s) distinguished the cases from the controls?
- What was the purpose of the study?
- What were the results of the study?

Table 6.1 | Examples of Cases and Controls in Cited Case-Control Studies

	Case	Control
Linens et al. (2014)	17 individuals with chronic ankle instability	17 healthy age-matched individuals without chronic ankle instability
Champagne et al. (2012)	15 older women with chronic low back pain	15 age-matched individuals with no back pain

functions related to balance. The study results indicated that older women with chronic low back pain had lower mobility scores that were related to lower scores on the balance confidence scale than older women without chronic low back pain.

Correlation and Prediction

Exploratory studies also frequently address correlation and prediction. A **correlational study** identifies the relationship, or degree of association, between variables. A **predictive study** is a type of correlational study that predicts an outcome based on the relationship between variables. These studies may also fall into other categories, such as retrospective or prospective, and cohort or case-control. The following examples demonstrate a variety of research designs.

Jijimol and associates (2013) conducted a prospective cohort study to determine whether trunk impairment is related to balance in patients with chronic stroke.[9] The correlational study included 30 participants who had previously been diagnosed with a stroke and who were able to sit with or without support. The participants were tested using a trunk impairment scale and the Tinetti balance scale. Scores on the two assessments were compared, and the results showed a strong correlation between the scores on the trunk impairment scale and the scores on the balance scale. This means that participants with less trunk impairment had better balance and participants with greater trunk impairment had poorer balance. The investigators' purpose for the study was simply to establish a relationship between trunk impairment and balance.

Weirich and associates (2010) conducted a prospective cross-sectional study to identify predictors of static and dynamic balance in women.[10] Three age categories were examined: young, identified as 18 to 25 years ($n = 30$); middle-aged, identified as 35 to 45 years ($n = 26$); and late middle-aged, identified as 55 to 64 ($n = 29$). They measured a variety of strength, flexibility, and anthropometric characteristics as well as static postural stability tests. The investigators identified one predictor of balance in young women, which was tandem walk sway velocity. They identified two predictors of balance in middle-aged women and five predictors for late middle-aged women, which included a variety of the static postural stability tests. This study went beyond identifying factors that were related to balance in order to identify factors that predicted balance.

Bland and associates (2012) conducted a retrospective cohort study to determine which admission clinical assessments would best predict a patient's discharge walking ability in a stroke inpatient rehabilitation facility setting.[11] Discharge walking ability was defined in the study as 10-meter walk speed. The predictive study was also set up to determine a clinical decision rule that would differentiate between household and community ambulators at discharge. A **clinical decision rule** is a combination of findings that have demonstrated meaningful predictability in determining a specific condition or diagnosis. The investigators reviewed medical records of patients who had previously been admitted to the inpatient rehabilitation facility during a 10-month period. Records of 227 participants were screened, but only 110 records included all of the measurements identified for the study. One of the disadvantages listed for retrospective studies was that records might not include all of the data points being investigated. Results from those 110 records showed that the Berg Balance Scale score and the walking score of the Functional Independence Measure were best able to predict discharge walking speed. The investigators also identified cut-off scores on those two measures (Berg Balance Scale score of ≤20, FIM walking score of 1 or 2) that would distinguish between household and community ambulators at discharge.

Methodological Research

Another type of exploratory research is called methodological research. Methodological research includes studies that are designed to develop measuring instruments for use in clinical practice and in research.[1,2] Part of the development process for a new instrument is testing to determine validity and reliability. Validity is the soundness or accuracy of a conclusion or measurement—in other words, the instrument measures what it is supposed to measure. Reliability is the ability to produce the same results in repeated measures when the conditions are the same—in other words, the measurement can be repeated with the same results. In methodological research, the instrument being developed must be compared with a well-established reference standard, sometimes called a gold standard, for validity to be determined. A gold standard is the test that is commonly accepted as the best available measure. For example, tests that assess range of motion of a joint can be compared with an x-ray image. As outcomes have become more important in clinical practice, the need for good outcome measuring instruments has gained importance. Let's look at some examples of methodological research.

Miyamoto and associates (2008) conducted a cross-sectional prospective study to develop a new agility performance test for elderly people.[12] The study was designed to assess the reliability and validity of the test that had been developed by the investigators. The authors suggested that agility was a component of motor function that was not being addressed adequately in performance tests used to determine risk for falling. The study included 828 healthy participants ranging in age from 20 to 99 years old, who were grouped according to age ranges. Participants were assessed using the new agility performance test, called the Ten Step Test, as well as several other standard tests. All participants older than 70 years were also asked whether they had fallen in the past year. To determine reliability, the same examiner conducted all of the tests, and each participant was measured in the Ten Step Test twice in the same day. A small number of participants also came back 1 week later to be retested. To determine validity, small subgroups of participants were also assessed using other tests that included a component of agility. The investigators determined that their Ten Step Test was a reliable measure of agility that could help predict risk for falling in elderly people.

Investigators may design a methodological study to determine the validity and reliability of an instrument that has been modified in some way from the original or is being used with a different type of patient or setting. The next example is a methodological study that was conducted by Forsberg and Nilsagard in 2013.[13] The purpose of their study was to determine the validity and reliability of the Swedish version of the Activities-specific Balance Confidence Scale (ABC scale) in patients with chronic stroke. The original ABC scale was in English, and the authors noted that a Swedish translation of the ABC scale had already been validated in more acute phases of stroke. The study included 67 community-dwelling participants who were at least 1 year post-stroke and were able to walk 10 meters independently. As with most self-assessment questionnaires, individuals were excluded who had difficulty understanding the language of the document, which in this case was Swedish. Participants were tested using the Swedish-version ABC scale as well as other standard balance and functional mobility tests commonly used in individuals with stroke. Participants were also asked if they had fallen within the past 3 months. One week after the assessment, another Swedish-version ABC scale was mailed to the participants. Validity was determined by comparing the results of the ABC scale with the results of the other tests, and the results showed significant correlations. Reliability was determined by comparing the ABC scale test and retest results on both individual questions and the overall score. The investigators concluded that the Swedish version of the ABC scale was a reliable and valid measure for determining balance confidence in individuals who are at least 1 year post-stroke.

Learning Task

Using PubMed, locate a methodological research article published during the past 10 years. Read the article and answer the following questions:

- What type of measuring instrument is being studied?
- Did the authors develop a new instrument, or did the authors apply an existing instrument to a new population of subjects?
- Did the article address the validity of the measuring instrument?
- Did the article address the reliability of the measuring instrument?

Addressing Biases and Threats

The information provided in this chapter regarding exploratory research should be helpful to the reader in reviewing and understanding the literature. Exploratory research is a useful tool and can often provide information that could not reasonably be collected in an experimental study. It is therefore important for the reader to understand the strengths and limitations of exploratory research. Let's review some of the strengths and limitations within exploratory research and compared with experimental research.

What are some reasons that an investigator might choose to use an exploratory design? A researcher may be interested in understanding how specific factors or characteristics interact with the environment without any manipulation of those factors. This is an underlying rationale in studies with a purpose of developing diagnostic and prognostic tests and measures. Or a researcher may be interested in developing a new way to measure characteristics or outcomes and determining whether the new measure is valid and reliable. As we saw in a couple of our examples, researchers were interested in identifying risk factors for falls. Such information would be helpful to clinicians to identify patients at risk for falling and possibly prevent future falls.

Sample Selection

Just as with experimental research, the clinician must be able to identify factors that could introduce bias or threaten the validity or quality of the study. One factor to be considered is the selection of the sample. The study must clearly identify the point at which participants were brought into the study (e.g., postoperative day 1, at least 6 months following a stroke, first day of spring training) as well as a common characteristic or impairment relevant to the study.[3] In our example of a prospective cohort study investigating fall rates, participants were admitted to the study when they were initially admitted to a facility for therapy, and the common characteristic was being elderly. Diagnosis was not a consideration for the study because the investigators wanted to include all elderly patients admitted for rehabilitation. In our first example of a prospective case-control study, the common impairment was chronic ankle instability. The investigators did not include participants with acute or subacute ankle injuries due to instability because that was not their population of interest. If they had included participants ranging from acute to chronic ankle instability, the results would likely have been different. In reviewing a study, the clinician must be able to identify the characteristics of the participants in order to determine whether the information is useful for their particular clinical question. It may be helpful to review the inclusion and exclusion criteria of a study to help identify the common factors used to develop the sample.

Tests and Measures

Another important consideration is the outcome measure or measures used and the point at which outcome measures were obtained. A research report should clearly explain why a particular measure or measures were selected. The report should also identify how the validity and reliability of the outcome measure was determined. The report should define when the outcome measures were used (e.g., admission to the rehabilitation facility, discharge from the hospital, 1 week after concluding a therapy episode of care). In the example of a prospective cohort correlational study, the report indicated that participants were tested on the trunk impairment scale and the Tinetti balance scale on the same day. The scores were then compared to see if there was a correlation between scores. If some participants completed both tests on the same day and some participants completed the tests 2 weeks apart, do you think the results might have been different?

Time Frame

An additional consideration is the length of the study. The time frame for the study needs to be long enough to ensure that the outcome of interest can be captured. Impairments such as a stroke may require months or even years before an individual's full functional potential is reached. If the purpose of a study is to investigate the ability of a stroke patient to achieve independence within the community, a time frame of 3 months would not be adequate. A study investigating the impact of a diet and exercise regimen on percentage of body fat would need to encompass enough time for the physiological changes to occur.

Comparison to Experimental Research

Some of the potential threats to validity that we discussed for experimental research also exist for exploratory research, such as small sample size or lack of blinding. Typically, sample sizes for exploratory studies are larger than for experimental studies, particularly for studies that are developing diagnostic or prognostic tests. A sample size that is too small can cause the reader to question whether the results are meaningful. Blinding is also important in exploratory research for the same reasons we identified in the previous chapter. Whenever possible, the individual collecting the data should not be the same person who is analyzing the data. In addition, the individual collecting the data should not be aware of the purpose of the study or the grouping of the participant. A study designed to develop a new test or measure should always compare the new test or measure to a reference standard, and participants must be tested using both measures. The individuals conducting the new test or measure should be blinded to the results of the reference testing. The testers should also be blinded to the patient's clinical information and history to ensure objectivity.

As with experimental research, it is important that the investigators use appropriate statistical tests when analyzing the data collected during a study. If an investigator uses the wrong statistical procedure to analyze the results, the conclusions may not be valid. A detailed discussion of statistical tests is beyond the scope of this textbook. However, peer review can assist the reader in feeling confident that the statistical analysis is likely appropriate for the data collected. Clinicians will become more familiar with statistical analysis as they become more experienced in reviewing and appraising the literature.

Application to Evidence Based Practice

A clinician should be able to identify the type of exploratory research as well as the type of research design. A clinician should also be able to determine whether a research design seems to be appropriate for answering the research question. Sometimes this can be as simple as deciding whether the research design "makes sense." As an example, a study specifically designed to determine the reliability of a newly developed testing procedure could not be designed as a retrospective study. Physical therapists (PTs) and physical therapist assistants (PTAs) should be able to determine the quality of evidence provided by exploratory research articles. They should be able to identify potential sources of bias and threats and determine whether the investigators addressed them adequately. Exploratory research is utilized for a variety of reasons, including diagnostic and prognostic studies and methodological research. Although diagnosis and prognosis are outside the role of the PTA, the PTA should be knowledgeable about factors that contribute to a diagnosis or prognosis. PTAs should also be able to utilize methodological research in the role of conducting selected data collection using reliable and valid tools. Exploratory research plays an important role in expanding the evidence base in physical therapy and provides a resource for the PT or PTA involved in evidence based practice.

SUMMARY

This chapter has covered various types of exploratory research that are commonly encountered during a review of the literature. Common types of exploratory research include cohort studies, case-control studies, correlation or prediction studies, and methodological research. A study can be designed to be retrospective (gathering data that has already been collected) or prospective (moving forward to collect data), and it can be designed to be longitudinal (following subjects over a long period of time) or cross-sectional (looking across groups at one point in time). Exploratory research investigates the relationships between variables and may attempt to predict whether a change in one variable can predict a change in another variable. Exploratory research can be used for the development of a diagnostic test or measure, to compare variables across categories, or to determine the incidence or history of a condition. Table 6.2 provides a summary of the examples cited in this chapter and reflects a variety of research designs commonly seen in exploratory research.

Table 6.2 | Summary of Cited Articles Reflecting a Variety of Research Designs

Study	Prospective	Retrospective	Longitudinal	Cross-Sectional
Morrison et al. (2011): Changes in fall risk factors	X		X	
Teasell et al. (2002): Falls in stroke patients		X		
Linens et al. (2014): Identifying individuals with chronic ankle instability	X			X
Champagne et al. (2012): Balance and fear avoidance with low back pain	X			X
Jijimol et al. (2013): Trunk impairment and balance in patients with stroke	X			X
Weirich et al. (2010): Predictors of static and dynamic balance	X			X

Table 6.2 | Summary of Cited Articles Reflecting a Variety of Research Designs—cont'd

Study	Prospective	Retrospective	Longitudinal	Cross-Sectional
Bland et al. (2012): Predictors of patient's discharge walking ability following stroke		X	X	
Miyamoto et al. (2008): Development of agility test for elderly people	X			X
Forsberg & Nilsagard (2013): Validity and Reliability of Swedish ABC Scale	X			X

● Case Scenario

You are going to be interviewing for a PTA position in a large teaching hospital, and your interview is scheduled for next week. In preparing for the interview, you noticed on the website that the therapy department is actively involved in several research studies. You want to appear knowledgeable about the facility and department for which you are applying, so you read about the studies being conducted. One of the studies is investigating the relationship between patient compliance, patient attitudes about therapy, patient satisfaction, and patient functional outcomes. The research design includes the use of admission patient questionnaires to determine patient attitudes, as well as patient satisfaction and compliance in general with their health-care practitioners before therapy. At the end of the therapy episode of care, the patient attitude questionnaire will be readministered, and a questionnaire to determine patient satisfaction and compliance with therapy will be administered. Therapists will administer a functional outcome measure at the beginning and end of therapy. Data are being collected over a 1-year period.

CASE QUESTIONS

Would this study be categorized as a:
1. Cohort study or a case-control study?

2. Longitudinal or cross-sectional study?

3. Retrospective or prospective study?

4. Correlational, predictive, or methodological study?

Review Activities

1. In your own words, explain the difference between a longitudinal study and a cross-sectional study.

   _____

   _____

   _____

   _____

2. In your own words, explain the difference between a cohort study and a case-control study.

   _____

   _____

   _____

   _____

3. Briefly explain the difference between independent groups design and repeated measures designs.

   _____

   _____

   _____

   _____

4. Identify the purpose of (a) a correlational study and (b) a predictive study.

   _____

   _____

   _____

   _____

5. Briefly discuss the importance of methodological research.

   _____

   _____

   _____

   _____

6. List three examples of threats to the validity of an exploratory study.

_____

_____

_____

_____

MATCHING

_____ 1. Predictive study   A. Subjects with condition being investigated

_____ 2. Correlational study   B. Collects new data

_____ 3. Longitudinal study   C. Study to identify relationship between variables

_____ 4. Cross-sectional study   D. Study follows specific group of subjects

_____ 5. Retrospective study   E. Subjects who do not have condition being studied

_____ 6. Prospective study   F. Study that predicts outcome based on relationship between variables

_____ 7. Cohort study   G. Study follows subjects over time with repeated measures

_____ 8. Case-control study   H. Study that compares subjects who do and do not have a certain condition

_____ 9. Cases   I. Study investigates subjects at one point in time

_____ 10. Controls   J. Investigation of data already collected

▮ References

1. Portney LG, Watkins MP. *Foundations of Clinical Research: Applications to Practice.* Upper Saddle River, NJ: Pearson Education; 2008.
2. Research Methods Knowledge Base. http://www.socialresearchmethods.net/kb/index.php. Accessed July 10, 2015.
3. Fetters L, Tilson J. *Evidence Based Physical Therapy.* Philadelphia, PA: F. A. Davis; 2012.
4. Barron J, Guidon M. Grip strength and functional balance in community-dwelling older women. *Int J Ther Rehabil.* 2011;18(11):622-630.
5. Morrison G, Lee H, Kuys SS, Clarke J, Bew P, Haines TP. Changes in fall risk factors for geriatric diagnostic groups across inpatient, outpatient and domiciliary rehabilitation settings. *Disabil Rehabil.* 2011;33(11):900-907.
6. Teasell R, McRae M, Foley N, Bhardwaj A. The incidence and consequences of falls in stroke patients during inpatient rehabilitation: factors associated with high risk. *Arch Phys Med Rehabil.* 2002;83:329-333.

7. Linens SW, Ross SE, Arnold BL, Gayle R, Pidcoe P. Postural-stability tests that identify individuals with chronic ankle instability. *J Athl Train.* 2014;49(1):15-23.

8. Champagne A, Prince F, Bouffard V, Lafond D. Balance, falls-related self-efficacy, and psychological factors amongst older women with chronic low back pain: a preliminary case-control study. *Rehabil Res Pract.* 2012; Article ID 430374, 8 pages.

9. Jijimol G, Fayaz RK, Vijesh PV. Correlation of trunk impairment with balance in patients with chronic stroke. *Neuro Rehabil.* 2013;32:323-325.

10. Weirich G, Bemben DA, Bemben MG. Predictors of balance in young, middle-aged, and late middle-aged women. *J Geriatr Phys Ther.* 2010;33(3):110-117.

11. Bland MD, Sturmoski A, Whitson M, et al. Prediction of discharge walking ability from initial assessment in a stroke inpatient rehabilitation facility population. *Arch Phys Med Rehabil.* 2012;93:1441-1447.

12. Miyamoto K, Takebayashi H, Takimoto K, Miyamoto S, Morioka S, Yagi F. A new simple performance test focused on agility in elderly people: the Ten Step Test. *Gerontol.* 2008;54:365-372.

13. Forsberg A, Nilsagard Y. Validity and reliability of the Swedish version of the Activities-specific Balance Confidence Scale in people with chronic stroke. *Physiother Can.* 2013;62(2):141-147.

Descriptive Research

Chapter at a Glance

Learning Outcomes

After reading this chapter, the reader will be able to:

· Discuss various types of descriptive research.
· Identify the role of normative research in physical therapy practice.
· List and define examples of qualitative research.
· Explain the purpose of a case study and a case series.
· Discuss the application of descriptive research to evidence based practice.

Key Terms

· Case series
· Case study
· Descriptive research
· Descriptive survey
· Developmental research
· Ethnography
· Grounded theory
· Likert scale
· Phenomenology

◘ FOOD FOR THOUGHT

You are a physical therapist assistant in a skilled nursing facility, and you are working with a 76-year-old man with a diagnosis of Parkinson disease. His symptoms have worsened in recent months, including his resting tremor and festinating gait. You have tried several treatment strategies to improve the quality of his gait, but he has shown minimal progress. You just received your new *Physical Therapy* journal and notice a case study about gait in a patient with Parkinson disease. You read the case report and notice that the patient in the case study is similar to your patient. The author of the case study describes a new type of walker specifically designed for patients with Parkinson disease, as well as a unique treatment intervention to improve a festinating gait.

Questions to consider:

· Would this information be useful to you?
· Would you try the treatment intervention described in the case study with your patient? Why or why not?

Introduction

This chapter will provide an explanation of descriptive research and examples of various types of research categorized as descriptive. The purpose of this chapter is to prepare the reader to critically appraise descriptive research articles during a literature search. **Descriptive research** is defined as research that is used to describe characteristics of a population or phenomenon.[1,2] This type of research can be used to describe what exists, categorize information, or determine the frequency of an occurrence. Types of descriptive research include normative research, qualitative research, developmental research, descriptive surveys, and case studies. Descriptive research may also overlap somewhat with exploratory research.[1] Descriptive research is commonly used as the beginning point for further research. For example, an investigator who is interested in a new treatment technique might conduct a case study with a single patient. The case study, including patient outcomes, could then lay the foundation for an exploratory or experimental study.

Normative Research

You are working in a clinic and measure your 65-year-old patient's knee flexion range of motion. How does your patient's range of motion compare with that of other individuals in the same age category? You might have seen a chart in a textbook that listed normal knee flexion range of motion for patients in various age categories (Table 7.1). The information in such a table would have been obtained through normative research. *Normative research* is defined as research that is designed to obtain and describe typical values for characteristics of a given population.[1-3] Normative data are important because they allow the clinician to identify areas in which a patient's measurement or outcome falls outside of values that are considered normal. The population may be defined by factors such as age, gender, or disability. In normative research, the investigator must clearly define the study population as well as the characteristic being measured. As outcome measures are developed, normative studies are critical to establishing standards to guide interpretation of the test results. Normative research requires large random samples to ensure that the results are truly characteristic of the population. It is also useful when multiple studies have investigated the same characteristics because similar results can validate the findings. Let's look at a couple of examples related to physical therapy practice.

Table 7.1 | Hip and Knee Motions: Mean Values in Degrees*

Author	Waugh et al.	Drews et al.	Schwarze and Denton	Wanatabe et al.	Phelps et al.	Booze and Azen	Roach and Miles	AAOS	AMA
	6–65 hr	12 hr–6 days	1–3 days	4 wk	9 mo	1–54 yr	25–74 yr		
	n = 40	n = 54	n = 1000	n = 62	n = 25	n = 109	n = 1,683		
Motion		(26 M, 26 F)	(473 M, 527 F)		(M and F)	(109 M)	(821 M, 862 F)		
Hip									
Flexion	–	–	–	138	–	122	121	120	100
Extension	46*	28*†	20*	12*	10*	10	19	20	30
Abduction	–	55‡	78‡	51	–	46	42		40
Adduction	–	6‡	15‡	–	–	27	–		20
Medial rotation	–	80‡	58	24	52	47	32	45	50
Lateral rotation	–	114‡	80	66	47	47	32	45	50
Knee									
Flexion	–	–	150	–	–	142	132	135	150
Extension	15*	20*	15*	–	–	–	–	10	–

† Tested with subjects in side-lying position.
‡ Tested with subjects in supine position.
AAOS, American Association of Orthopaedic Surgeons; AMA, American Medical Association; F, females; M, males.
Source: Norkin CC, White DJ. *Measurement of Joint Motion: A Guide to Goniometry.* 4th ed. Philadelphia: F. A. Davis; 2009, with permission.

O'Hoski and associates (2014) identified a need for age-related normative scores on an outcome measure for balance called the Balance Evaluation Systems Test (BESTest), as well as two shorter versions of the same test.[4] The BESTest was developed for individuals with Parkinson disease, and earlier studies demonstrated good reliability and validity for the test in patients with Parkinson disease. The investigators planned to identify age-related normative scores on all three tests in healthy individuals by age category, which would provide clinicians with data to compare patient results with age-matched normal results. The study included 79 participants ranging in age from 50 to 89 years, and participants were categorized by age decade (50 to 59, 60 to 69, 70 to 79, and 80 to 89 years). Each participant completed the BESTest, and scores were then determined for the BEST, the mini-BEST, and the brief-BESTest. The study results demonstrated that balance scores showed a significant decline with age and also revealed greater variability in scores as age increased. The authors noted that their sample size was not large enough for the results to be generalized to all populations, and they indicated a need for further normative study in the 50- to 89-year age range as well as other ages.

Another study documented sex- and age-specific normative values for steps per day for older adults.[5] The data were collected from the National Health and Nutrition Examination Survey (NHANES) and included 1,196 participants who were aged 60 years and older. (Note the much larger sample size than the previous study.) The investigators categorized participants by 5-year age ranges (e.g., 60 to 64, 65 to 69 years). Data for the NHANES were collected using an accelerometer, so the authors adjusted the data to a pedometer scale because pedometers are more commonly used in clinical and health/wellness settings. The results of the study revealed that steps per day tended to decrease as age category increased. Men aged >65 to 69 years represented the category with the highest number of steps per day (<9,126 steps/day), whereas women aged 85+ years represented were the category with the lowest number of steps (@276 steps/day). The authors presented the results in a table format to allow clinicians to make quick comparisons of patient results to the normal values. Because of the relationship between physical activity and health in aging adults, the data from this study can assist the clinician in identifying patients who fall outside of normal values for age and gender.

Learning Task

Using PubMed, locate a normative study related to physical therapy. Read the article and answer the following questions:

• What was the characteristic being measured?
• How big was the sample size?
• Do you think the sample size was adequate?
• What were the group parameters and how many groups were used?
• Would this information be useful to you in providing patient care?

Qualitative Research

Another type of descriptive research is qualitative research. Qualitative research is defined as research that emphasizes the individual perspective by describing aspects of human nature and an individual's perception of their own experiences. As noted by Portney and Watkins, qualitative research goes beyond describing a situation by attempting to understand, explain, or develop a theory about an observed phenomenon.[1] Qualitative research differs from quantitative research in several ways (Table 7.2). Qualitative research uses subjects' words and narrative as data, rather than numbers, and will typically include direct quotes made within the research report. Qualitative research emphasizes discussion and debate of hypotheses rather than conclusions and final results. And finally, qualitative research includes the researcher as an important part of the investigation. In quantitative research, every effort is made to remove the researcher from data collection, such as through blinding/masking.

Table 7.2 | Comparison of Quantitative and Qualitative Research Paradigms*

	Quantitative	Qualitative
Assumption	Single objective reality	Multiple realities
Purpose	To test, verify, or predict	To describe in detail or explain
Designs	Experimental or observational	Ethnography, case study
Methods	Controlled interventions	Observation, interview
Data	Quantitative, statistical analysis	Qualitative, words, documents

Source: Hack L, Gwyer J. *Evidence into Practice: Integrating Judgment, Values, and Research.* Philadelphia: F. A. Davis; 2013, with permission.

Qualitative research should be considered an important component of evidence based practice because it can assist the clinician in understanding the dynamics of the patient perspective. Although qualitative research is often overlooked by clinicians, it can be an important tool in evidence based practice. Qualitative research should be carefully conducted using clear sampling strategies, a methodical data analysis, and a commitment by the investigators to examine alternative explanations. Green and Britten (1998) noted that qualitative research can "bridge the gap" between evidence and practice and may help clinicians understand barriers to using evidence in certain patient circumstances.[6]

Several different approaches can be used for qualitative research. The most commonly used approaches are phenomenology, grounded theory, and ethnography. **Phenomenology** is defined as a method of explaining complex phenomena by analyzing narrative information provided by individual subjects and identifying themes. As an example, Greenfield and associates conducted a study to explore the meaning of caring from the perspective of the novice physical therapist (PT).[7] They interviewed seven PTs who had been practicing less than a year. The investigators identified three common themes that emerged, including learning to care, patients as subjects, and the culture of the clinic. The clinicians revealed that learning to care included challenges such as time management—allowing time to listen to and talk with patients—and dealing with difficult patients. The clinicians also consistently noted that the values and behaviors of other therapists in the clinic influenced how they cared for their patients.

Grounded theory is another approach to qualitative research. **Grounded theory** involves the discovery of theory through the analysis of data; in other words, the theory is "grounded" in the data. This differs from more typical research methods that begin with a theory, then collect data to support or refute the theory. An example of grounded theory is a study by Barnsley and associates.[8] The investigators explored the experiences and attitudes of individuals with stroke who traveled outdoors soon after hospital discharge. The study included 19 subjects who had been hospitalized following a stroke and were still receiving rehabilitation on an outpatient basis. The researchers conducted interviews with the subjects as well as eight significant others. They categorized subjects as either hesitant or confident explorers based on walking, using public transportation, and driving. The researchers identified factors that influenced outdoor travel, including emotional state, meaningful destinations, expectations for recovery, and social network. Subjects who had a walking habit before a stroke were more likely to be confident explorers. "Gatekeepers" had a negative impact on outdoor travel when subjects perceived that they should not walk outdoors, cross streets, and so forth because of restrictions set by health-care professionals or family members.

Ethnography is another commonly seen methodology in qualitative research. **Ethnography** is the study of attitudes, beliefs, and behaviors of a culture through observation of individuals within their own setting. Cultures may be defined fairly broadly to include groups of individuals within a profession, a work setting, or other social organizational structure. A study by Thompson explored the social meaning and function of humor in physical therapy practice by observing and interviewing therapists in the clinical setting.[9] The investigator spent time with the subjects over a 6-month period of time and identified patterns of behavior within the team's culture. Humor was used by the more senior therapist as a management tool to deal with minor transgressions and encourage the team to use particular strategies. Humor was used by the team members to build relationships and promote the concept of team.

Developmental Research

Another type of descriptive research is developmental research. **Developmental research** involves describing developmental behaviors and the normal sequence and changes over time. Developmental studies can be longitudinal or cross-sectional in design. A longitudinal study would require the investigator to make repeated observations of the same individuals over time. In a cross-sectional study, the researcher would investigate a group of subjects categorized by age levels at one point in time. Developmental research often forms the foundation for exploratory or experimental research.

An example of developmental research can be found in a study by Marsala and VanSant published in 1998.[10] The researchers conducted a cross-sectional study to describe the movement patterns of toddlers when moving from a supine position to a standing position. The study included 60 children between the ages of 15 and 47 months. The researchers were able to describe the movement patterns by age categories and identify age-related differences.

A second example of developmental research published in 2014 investigated the differences in gray and white brain matter volume in school-aged children with speech sound errors.[11] The study included 23 children identified with speech sound errors and 54 children without speech sound errors that were matched for age, IQ, and oral language. The investigators were able to describe brain gray and white matter volumes in specific areas of the brain at different ages for children with and without speech sound errors.

Descriptive Surveys

Surveys are a commonly used tool in research. A specific type of survey that can be classified as descriptive research is the descriptive survey. A **descriptive survey** is designed to gather data to describe the characteristics, behaviors, or attitudes of a particular group.[1] Descriptive surveys may be cross-sectional or longitudinal in nature. Questions on a survey may be closed-ended questions, in which respondents choose from multiple choices provided on the survey tool, or open-ended questions, in which choices are not provided and respondents must provide an answer to a question. Let's look at a couple of examples.

Biddiss and associates (2011) conducted an international survey study to investigate the impact of prosthetic cost and funding on the use of upper limb prosthetics.[12] The investigators developed a survey tool that used a combination of open-ended questions, closed-ended questions, and 4- and 5-point Likert scale ratings. A **Likert scale** is a scale designed to allow respondents to identify their level of agreement or disagreement with an item in order to capture the intensity of perceptions or feelings. Figure 7.1 provides an example of a Likert scale. Responses to the survey ($n = 242$) indicated that access to funding for prosthetics varied by age, country, and level of limb loss. Of the individuals who reported on costs ($n = 109$), 37% indicated that they were financially disadvantaged by both the initial costs and ongoing maintenance costs. Of the nonprosthetic wearers ($n = 71$), about half indicated that cost was an important factor in their decision not to use a prosthetic. The investigators were able to provide clinicians with important patient considerations for working with individuals with amputations.

A second example of a descriptive survey study investigated the practice patterns and beliefs of hand therapists in treating acute and chronic lateral epicondylitis.[13] The investigators developed a survey tool that used both open-ended and closed-ended questions. The results of the survey responses were compiled, and responses were

Indicate the degree to which you agree with the following statements using the scale below.

1 = Strongly agree	**2** = Agree	**3** = Neither agree nor disagree
	4 = Disagree	**5** = Strongly disagree

	1	**2**	**3**	**4**	**5**
Every PT and PTA should be involved in providing pro bono services.	❑	❑	❑	❑	❑
Every individual in the U.S. should have access to PT services.	❑	❑	❑	❑	❑

Figure 7.1 An example of a 5-point Likert scale. A Likert scale allows respondents to identify their level of agreement or disagreement with an item in order to capture the intensity of perceptions or feelings.

ranked in order of frequency. The researchers were able to identify the most commonly used examination and diagnostic techniques for both acute and chronic lateral epicondylitis, as well as the most commonly used treatments and outcome measures. The investigators were able to provide clinicians with information about the range of interventions and other tools used by hand therapists in treating this diagnosis.

Case Studies

Another type of descriptive research is the case study. A **case study** is a detailed description of an individual patient or client and the outcomes of the case. A case study can also address a group, such as a family, or an institution, such as a physical therapy program or department. A case study is essentially a description of practice and cannot be generalized to other patients. A **case series** is similar to a case study but includes multiple cases with similar diagnoses or circumstances. Case studies and case series frequently address interesting or unique patient problems or diagnoses and will typically include diagnoses, history, behaviors, assessment, interventions, and outcomes. Case studies are important to clinicians as a means of expanding their clinical knowledge base beyond patient experiences they have encountered first-hand. They also serve to generate ideas, hypotheses, or techniques that can be followed up later with experimental research. Portney and Watkins identified several purposes for case studies, including understanding unusual patient conditions, providing examples of innovative or creative therapies, generating and testing a theory, and providing direction for future research.[1] Figure 7.2 depicts the difference between a case study and a case series. Let's look at some examples of case studies and case series in physical therapy.

Scibek and Carcia (2012) presented a case study about a 41-year-old man with a diagnosis of acute calcific tendinopathy.[14] They described the results of a conservative treatment approach that included superficial modalities and medications for pain along with a therapeutic exercise program. The authors compared this approach to other documented treatments for the same diagnosis that included ultrasound, diathermy, shock-wave therapy, steroid injections, and surgery. The case study included a detailed account of the initial onset of symptoms, assessment by multiple health care professionals, radiographic results, and various unique aspects of the case. The authors described the excellent patient outcomes followed by a lengthy discussion about the diagnosis, treatment, and unique aspects of the case. They noted that the unique aspects of this case were different from those of other cases with a similar diagnosis that had been presented in the literature.

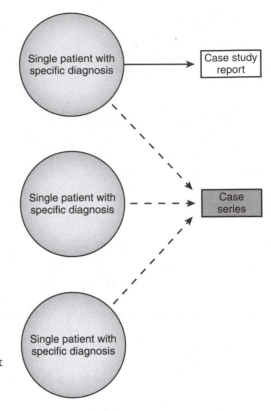

Figure 7.2 A comparison of a case study and a case series. Each patient included in a case series must have the same diagnosis or condition.

The next example is a case study about a single physical therapy program. The purpose of the case study was to describe a unique workload model for faculty in a physical therapy program and the outcomes of model implementation.[15] The authors noted that faculty members in physical therapy programs are expected to teach, advise students, participate in research activities, and participate in clinical practice. Faculty members at the program in the case study were assigned more responsibilities related to teaching, with too little emphasis placed on research activities and clinical practice. The workload model was revised to consider all of the responsibilities for faculty, and faculty productivity increased as a result. Faculty had more time to participate in research and clinical practice without any impact on the student educational experience. The authors presented the case study to contribute to the literature regarding faculty workload and faculty expectations.

An example of a case series described the effects of cognitive-behavioral-based physical therapy in patients with a fear of moving following spinal surgery.[16] The case series included eight patients who had all undergone lumbar spine surgery for a degenerative condition. All eight patients completed the same therapy intervention and completed the same performance-based outcome measures. The investigators reported that all eight patients had significant reduction of disability at their 6-month follow-up, and seven patients had significant reduction in pain. The researchers indicated that, although the case series provided preliminary data on the feasibility of this type of therapy, a randomized clinical trial would be needed to verify their results.

Another example of a case series published in 2014 described the treatment of three patients with Parkinson disease using a technique called Lee Silverman Voice Treatment Big (LSVT BIG).[17] The treatment technique consists of an intense program of high-amplitude movements. Each subject received 16 one-hour treatment sessions over a four-week period, and treatments were administered by two therapists who were certified in the LSVT BIG treatment method. All three individuals demonstrated improvement in a number of outcome measures related to gait, balance, and mobility. The investigators presented the case series to suggest that LSVT BIG may be beneficial for gait, balance, and bed mobility and suggested that further research using randomized controlled trials is needed to determine the effectiveness of this treatment technique.

Learning Task

Using CINAHL, locate a case study or case series related to physical therapy that was published during the past 5 years. Read the article and answer the following questions:

• What was the unique characteristic or treatment method being described?
• How many patients were included?
• Did the authors recommend further research on the topic being addressed?
• Would this information be useful to you in providing patient care?

Addressing Biases and Threats to Validity

The information provided in this chapter regarding descriptive research should be helpful to the reader in reviewing and understanding the literature. Descriptive research is a useful tool and can often serve as the basis for future exploratory or experimental study. It is therefore important for the reader to understand the strengths and limitations of descriptive research. Let's review some of the strengths and limitations within descriptive research and in comparison with exploratory and experimental research.

What are some reasons that an investigator might choose to use a descriptive design? A researcher may be interested in describing normal values for a particular characteristic, such as muscle strength or flexibility, in specified age categories. This is an underlying rationale in normative studies. An investigator may also desire to describe normal motor or cognitive development in a specific group or groups, which could be accomplished using developmental research. A researcher may be interested in taking a closer look at individuals' perspectives related to a particular phenomenon, which would involve a qualitative design. Clinicians may be interested in sharing information about a unique treatment technique that they believe will be helpful to other clinicians, which would be presented as a case study or case series.

Several aspects of descriptive research design are critical to ensuring the quality of the study. As with other types of research, the selection of the sample is important. The individuals selected for the study must be appropriate for the research question involved. For a normative study, the sample size must be sufficiently large to ensure that the results are truly characteristic of the population being described. The investigator must also clearly define the study population and the characteristic being measured. In developmental research, the investigator must also clearly define the age groups under investigation. Randomization is not used in descriptive research because this type of research does not include comparison groups.

Descriptive research is commonly used as a starting point for further research by describing what exists. Clearly, descriptive research is less rigorous than experimental or exploratory research, but it can be important in answering research questions related to developing an understanding of clinical phenomena. Descriptive research can also be used to answer research questions that would not fit into an experimental or exploratory design. In physical therapy, a need exists to describe many clinical behaviors or phenomena so that we can understand what exists. This can lay the foundation for beginning to explore relationships or cause and effect. As an example, a recent study assessed the normal values for timed static balance tests in school-aged children. The authors noted that static balance tests are commonly used to measure the balance abilities of children, but age-appropriate normative scores had not previously been identified.

Application to Evidence Based Practice

A clinician should be able to identify the type of descriptive research as well as the research design. A clinician should also be able to determine whether the research design is appropriate for answering the research question. The PT and physical therapist assistant (PTA) should be able to understand the strengths and limitations of descriptive research and determine the quality of evidence provided by descriptive research articles. Descriptive research is used for a variety of reasons, including normative research, developmental research, qualitative research, and case studies/case series. PTAs can use each of these types of research to expand their clinical knowledge and expertise. When collecting objective data on a patient, normative research is very helpful to compare patient results to the norm. When working with a pediatric patient with developmental or neurological impairment, developmental research is useful in understanding normal development as a comparison. Qualitative research can be very useful in helping the PTA better understand patient perceptions or patient circumstances. And finally, case studies or case series can enlighten the PTA about unique patient situations or unique treatment techniques that can be added to the clinician's bank of knowledge. Descriptive research plays an important role in evidence based practice for knowledgeable clinicians who understand the relevance of the different research designs.

SUMMARY

This chapter has covered various types of descriptive research that are commonly encountered during a review of the literature. Common types of descriptive research include normative research, developmental research, qualitative research, descriptive surveys, and case studies and case series. Normative research is designed to describe typical values for characteristics of a population. Qualitative research is designed to emphasize the individual perspective and perception of experiences. Developmental research is designed to describe developmental behaviors and the normal sequence and changes over time. Descriptive survey research is designed to describe the characteristics, behaviors, or attitudes of a particular group. Case studies and case series are designed to describe the details of an individual client or clients and typically address interesting or unique diagnoses or treatment techniques. Descriptive research is often used as the basis for future exploratory or experimental study.

● Case Scenario

You have recently begun working as a pediatric PTA in a small practice, and you are particularly interested in working with infants with torticollis and plagiocephaly. Your clinic works with a specialty clinic in a larger city that fits cranial remolding orthoses, or helmets, to reshape the infant's skull. You have reviewed the literature and are learning a lot about the two conditions, particularly the most current treatment interventions that are supported by research. However, you are curious about the impact of the diagnoses on the infant's families, particularly the parents. You have noticed that some parents seem to deal with the added stresses of their child's diagnosis and treatments without any difficulty, whereas other parents seem traumatized by the situation. You are very interested in finding some research that addresses the parent perspective with these diagnoses.

CASE QUESTIONS

1. What type of articles would you search for?

_____

_____

2. Which specific type of research would be best for this type of clinical question?

_____

_____

3. How likely do you think it is that you could find an article that addresses your specific question or interest?

_____

_____

Learning Task
Using any search tool, locate a descriptive research article that addresses torticollis, plagiocephaly, or the parent perspective in dealing with these diagnoses. Read your article and be prepared to participate in group discussion with classmates. Identify the research design and describe how it would apply to the case scenario.

Review Activities

1. Describe the purpose of a normative study and provide an example.

   _____

   _____

   _____

   _____

2. In your own words, describe the purpose of qualitative research and relevance to evidence based practice.

   _____

   _____

   _____

   _____

3. List strengths and weaknesses of case studies.

   _____

   _____

   _____

   _____

4. List two characteristics of case series.

   _____

   _____

   _____

   _____

MATCHING

_____ 1. Normative research	A. Study of a culture within its own setting
_____ 2. Phenomenology	B. Research method designed to gather data about characteristics of a group
_____ 3. Ethnography	C. Research that emphasizes individual perspective
_____ 4. Grounded theory	D. Research used to illustrate characteristics of a population
_____ 5. Developmental research	E. Research method for explaining complex occurrences

_____ 6. Qualitative research

F. Measurement scale that captures level of agreement or disagreement

_____ 7. Descriptive research

G. Research that describes normal sequence over time

_____ 8. Likert scale

H. Research designed to obtain typical values for a specific population

References

1. Portney LG, Watkins MP. *Foundations of Clinical Research: Applications to Practice.* Upper Saddle River, NJ: Pearson Education; 2008.
2. Research Methods Knowledge Base. http://www.socialresearchmethods.net/kb/index.php. Accessed July 12, 2015.
3. Fetters L, Tilson J. *Evidence Based Physical Therapy.* Philadelphia, PA: F. A. Davis; 2012.
4. O'Hoski S, Winship B, Herridge L, et al. Increasing the clinical utility of the BESTest, Mini-BESTest, and Brief-BESTest: normative values in Canadian adults who are healthy and aged 50 years or older. *Phys Ther.* 2014;94(3):334-342.
5. Tudor-Locke C, Schuna JM, Barreira TV, et al. Normative steps/day values for older adults: NHANES 2005-2006. *J Gerontol A Biol Sci Med Sci.* 2013;68(11):1426-1432.
6. Green J, Britten N. Qualitative research and evidence based medicine. *Br Med J.* 1998;316:1230-1232.
7. Greenfield BH, Anderson A, Cox B, Tanner MC. Meaning of caring to 7 novice physical therapists during their first year of clinical practice. *Phys Ther.* 2008; 88(10):1154-1166.
8. Barnsley L, McCluskey A, Middleton S. What people say about travelling outdoors after their stroke: a qualitative study. *Aust Occup Ther J.* 2012;59:71-78.
9. Thompson D. The social meaning and function of humour in physiotherapy practice: an ethnography. *Physiother Theory Pract.* 2010;26(11):1-11.
10. Marsala G, VanSant AF. Age-related differences in movement patterns used by toddlers to rise from a supine position to erect stance. *Phys Ther.* 1998;78(2):149-159.
11. Preston JL, Molfese PJ, Mencl WE, et al. Structural brain differences in school-age children with residual speech sound errors. *Brain Lang.* 2014;128:25-33.
12. Biddiss E, McKeever P, Lindsay S, Chau T. Implications of prosthetic funding structures on the use of prostheses: experiences of individuals with upper limb absence. *Prosthet Orthot Int.* 2011;35(2):215-224.
13. MacDermid JC, Wojkowski S, Kargus C, Marley M, Stevenson E. Hand therapist management of the lateral epicondylitis: a survey of expert opinion and practice patterns. *J Hand Ther.* 2009;23:18-30.
14. Scibek J, Carcia C. Presentation and conservative management of acute calcific tendinopathy: a case study and literature review. *J Sport Rehabil.* 2012;21:334-342.
15. Keskula DC, Mishoe S, Wark ET. Redefining faculty workloads in a physical therapy department: a case study. *J Allied Health.* 2011;40(3):e49-e53.
16. Archer KR, Motzny N, Abraham CM, et al. Cognitive-behavioral-based physical therapy to improve spine outcomes: a case series. *Phys Ther.* 2013;93(8):1130-1139.
17. Janssens J, Malfroid K, Nyffeler T, Bohlhalter S, Vanbellingen T. Application of LSVT BIG intervention to address gait, balance, bed mobility, and dexterity in people with Parkinson Disease: a case series. *Phys Ther.* 2014;94:1014-1023.

Research Reviews and Clinical Practice Guidelines

Chapter at a Glance

Learning Outcomes

After reading this chapter, the reader will be able to:

· Discuss the difference between a systematic review and a meta-analysis.
· Describe the key characteristics of a systematic review and a meta-analysis.
· Explain the purpose and function of a clinical practice guideline.
· Identify the role of research reviews and clinical practice guidelines in physical therapy practice.

Key Terms

· Cochrane Collaboration
· Conference proceeding
· Power

◘ FOOD FOR THOUGHT

You are a new graduate physical therapist assistant (PTA) working in a general outpatient physical therapy clinic. You are hoping to attend a continuing education course related to low back pain because that diagnosis makes up a large percentage of patient diagnoses in the clinic. Your clinic provides a small amount of funding per year to attend continuing education, and you want to make sure your money is well spent. You look online and find three different courses being offered in your area in the next couple of months. The most expensive course is presented by an individual whose name you recognize from ads in some magazines you saw while you were in school.

The course description indicates that the techniques presented in the course have been developed by the speaker during 25 years of clinical experience working with low back pain. The second course being offered is a symposium with a variety of guest speakers who are all certified clinical specialists in orthopedic physical therapy. The course description indicates that the symposium will present the most current evidence based guidelines for treating low back pain. The least expensive course is a 1-day course focused on using a particular physical agent in the treatment of low back pain. The course description indicates that the speaker has been using the equipment for several years and will demonstrate how to incorporate the equipment into your clinical practice. The course is sponsored by a vendor of the equipment.

Questions to consider:

· Do you think the content of all three courses is supported by best evidence? Why or why not?

· As a new graduate, which course would be most beneficial to improving your knowledge and why?

Introduction

This chapter provides a discussion of research reviews and clinical practice guidelines. The purpose of this chapter is to prepare the reader to critically appraise research reviews and clinical practice guidelines during a literature search. Research reviews and clinical practice guidelines include reviews of original research along with an evaluation of the original reports. Research reviews include systematic reviews and meta-analyses of exploratory and experimental research, and they also include clinical practice guidelines. Research reviews are useful tools in helping clinicians manage the vast amounts of information available today and should be included in searches for evidence to address a clinical question. Most hierarchies of evidence place research reviews and clinical practice guidelines at or near the top of the hierarchy, meaning that they are the preferred types of evidence in evidence based practice.

This chapter will provide an overview of systematic reviews, meta-analyses, and clinical practice guidelines. To provide clarity for comparison of the different types of evidence, examples in this chapter will use reports that address orthopedic conditions. Table 8.1 provides a comparison of systematic reviews, meta-analyses, and clinical practice guidelines.

Systematic Reviews

A systematic review is a special type of study that applies the scientific method to a review of the literature. A systematic review is defined as "a rigorous process of searching, appraising, and summarizing existing information on a selected topic."[1] The review focuses on a specific research or clinical question and includes an assessment of the quality of studies selected and a synthesis of the results. A systematic review differs from a general literature review. A general literature review typically includes only a small part of the research evidence because the evidence is provided

Table 8.1 | Comparison of Articles Addressing Systematic Reviews, Meta-analyses, and Clinical Practice Guidelines

	Systematic Review	Meta-analysis	Clinical Practice Guideline
Authors	Individual(s)	Individual(s)	Typically a panel of experts
Purpose	Answer a specific research/clinical question	Answer a specific research/clinical question	Develop recommendations for diagnosis, treatment, or prevention of health problems
In-depth literature review	Required	Required	May be included
Defined inclusion and exclusion criteria	Yes	Yes	Likely
Assessment of quality of studies	Yes	Yes	Yes
Statistical analysis	No	Yes	Only if meta-analysis is conducted
Synthesis of findings	Yes	Yes	Yes

primarily as illustrative examples.[2] A systematic review is a comprehensive review that attempts to find as much as possible of the relevant research related to the particular question. The key characteristics of a systematic review are (1) clearly articulated objectives with eligibility criteria determined before the review; (2) a precise methodology that can be duplicated and updated; (3) an organized and methodical search that attempts to identify all relevant studies; (4) an appraisal of the validity of the studies' findings; and (5) an organized presentation and synthesis of the findings.[2] The systematic review article should address all of these characteristics, including search engines and databases, search terms, criteria for grading evidence, appraisal of selected studies, and a summary of findings.

The authors of a systematic review will develop a research question and outline the methodology of the study before they review the literature. Specific criteria will be identified to determine what studies will be included or excluded. The authors will conduct a thorough review of the literature, using an organized step-by-step approach, and will select studies that meet the criteria. Authors will also commonly review conference proceeding materials from conferences that might provide information relevant to their question. Conferences are a source of current research being conducted; investigators frequently report at conferences on research they are conducting and may solicit audience feedback. A **conference proceeding** is a published version of the papers and abstracts presented at a conference. Some of the research may be published as an article at a later date, and some of the research may never be published as an article. Most systematic reviews of intervention questions will focus on randomized controlled trials (RCTs), which are considered the gold standard for intervention research. The selected studies will be critically reviewed and analyzed, and the authors will present their findings. Let's look at a couple of examples related to total knee replacements. Both examples are from the Cochrane Collaboration Database of Systematic Reviews. The **Cochrane Collaboration** is a nonprofit organization in the United Kingdom that advocates evidence based decision-making and provides a database of evidence primarily geared toward systematic reviews and meta-analyses.[2]

The first example of a systematic review is "Cryotherapy Following Total Knee Replacement."[3] The authors described the purpose of the review, which was to evaluate the acute use of cryotherapy following total knee replacement on pain, blood loss, and function. The reviewers searched a number of databases to identify all published RCTs or controlled clinical trials in which the experimental group received any type of cryotherapy following a total knee replacement. The report included the search methodology and a description of the inclusion and exclusion criteria. The reviewers also examined the references of identified studies for possible additional studies and reviewed the conference proceedings from organizations that were likely to address the topics. Two reviewers worked independently to review search results, then compared and discussed their findings. If the primary reviewers were unable to agree, a third reviewer was used. The reviewers selected 12 RCTs and clinical trials that met their inclusion criteria, and the studies included a total of 809 subjects. The review identified low-quality evidence that cryotherapy had small benefit for the outcomes chosen, including blood loss, pain, and range of motion. The authors concluded that benefits were likely too small to justify cryotherapy use.

A second example of a systematic review investigated the literature regarding continuous passive motion (CPM) following a total knee replacement.[4] This review is actually an update of two earlier reviews from 2003 and 2010. The purpose of the review was to assess the benefits and harm of CPM following total knee replacement. The reviewers searched a number of databases to identify all published RCTs in which the experimental group received CPM following a total knee replacement, and both the experimental and the control group received similar care otherwise. Two reviewers worked independently to review search results, then compared and discussed their findings. The reviewers identified 684 articles from the searches and reviewed 62 potentially eligible trials. Of those potentially eligible, 24 RCTs met their inclusion criteria, and the studies included a total of 1,445 subjects. Four of the trials were new since the previous review in 2010. The reviewers found moderate- to low-quality evidence that CPM had no clinically important effects on knee range of motion, pain, function, or quality of life. They also found low- to very-low-quality evidence that CPM may reduce the risk for manipulation under anesthesia and the risk for adverse side effects. The authors concluded that benefits were likely too small to justify CPM use.

Although most systematic reviews search for RCTs or controlled clinical trials, they can also be conducted using different types of evidence. For example, a recent systematic review was conducted to review guidelines for the physical management of osteoarthritis.[5] The reviewers searched numerous databases to identify all guidelines, protocols, and recommendations for the management or treatment of osteoarthritis. They identified 17 guidelines that met the inclusion criteria, and the selected criteria were independently reviewed. The reviewers identified a total of 40 interventions that were recommended, with the strongest recommendations found for exercise and education. Other interventions that were supported by strong evidence included electrical-based therapy, equipment, diet and weight loss, manual therapy, and self-management. The reviewers noted that other interventions were either unsupported or not recommended, such as acupuncture, massage therapy, and aspects of psychosocial-based therapy. The reviewers concluded that exercise and education were among the strongest recommendations and also relatively cost-effective to provide.

Learning Task

Go to the Cochrane website (www.cochrane.org) and locate a systematic review related to an orthopedic condition that was published within the past 5 years. Read the article and answer the following questions:

• What question are the reviewers investigating?
• What are the inclusion and exclusion criteria?
• How many studies were initially located? How many were included in the review?
• How many subjects were included in all of the selected studies?
• What were the reviewers' conclusions?
• What was the level of evidence for each conclusion/recommendation?

Meta-analysis

A meta-analysis is a specific type of systematic review that includes a statistical analysis of the outcomes of selected studies. Meta-analysis refers to the statistical methods of combining or integrating the results of selected studies.[1,6] In a meta-analysis, the preliminary steps are the same as for other systematic reviews. Then the results of the studies that meet the criteria are combined and analyzed quantitatively using meta-analysis. In some instances, the reviewers may plan to conduct a meta-analysis, but the studies may not provide results that are similar enough or appropriate for meta-analysis. Meta-analysis has been referred to as "conducting research about research."[7] A meta-analysis can increase the power of a single-study analysis to determine whether the treatment effects across multiple studies are comparable in similar situations. **Power** is defined as the probability that a study will detect an intervention effect of a specified size that is statistically significant.[6] Combining several studies with small groups of subjects through meta-analysis can increase the pool of subjects and improve the power of the results. The studies must be similar in research design and outcome measures in order for the results to be combined and analyzed.

One example of a meta-analysis is, "Does Exercise Reduce Pain and Improve Physical Function Before Hip or Knee Replacement Surgery? A Systematic Review and Meta-Analysis of Randomized Controlled Trials."[8] The purpose of the meta-analysis was described by the reviewers as investigating the effectiveness of exercise in reducing pain and improving function before joint replacement surgery. Eighteen studies met the inclusion criteria for the review and meta-analysis. The data from the studies were pooled, and a statistical analysis was conducted. The researchers conducting the meta-analysis determined no significant differences between the exercise groups and the no-intervention groups (from multiple studies) for patients awaiting knee surgery but did find a significant difference between patients awaiting hip surgery. By combining results from the studies included in the review, the authors were able to provide an analysis of the treatment effects across multiple situations and increase the power of the results.

A second example of a meta-analysis investigated the efficacy of strengthening or aerobic exercise on pain relief in people with knee osteoarthritis.[9] The authors used a number of search tools to locate studies. RCTs were included, and observational studies were excluded. The studies selected included non-weight-bearing strengthening exercises, weight-bearing strengthening exercises, or aerobic exercises. The reviewers initially identified a total of 559 studies, but only 8 studies met the criteria. The pooled subject size was 466 participants, with the initial studies ranging in subject size from 20 to 102. The results revealed that muscle strengthening exercises (weight-bearing and non-weight-bearing) and aerobic exercise were all effective for pain relief in individuals with knee osteoarthritis. For pain relief from a short-term exercise program, non-weight-bearing strengthening exercises were the most effective.

Clinical Practice Guidelines

Clinical practice guidelines are evidence based recommendations for the diagnosis, treatment, or prevention of health-care problems that are typically developed by a panel of experts. The majority of clinical guidelines are developed through the funding of professional associations, government entities, or health-care organizations. Most clinical practice guidelines will include a systematic review of the literature followed by recommendations for clinical decision-making. The panel of experts provides clinical expertise in the review of evidence and the development of recommendations. Although similar to a systematic review, clinical practice guidelines are typically broader in scope. Let's look at a couple of examples.

The first example of a clinical guideline is, "Ottawa Panel Evidence-Based Clinical Practice Guidelines for Aerobic Walking Programs in the Management of Osteoarthritis."[10] The Ottawa Panel was a group of Canadian researchers selected to produce evidence based clinical practice guidelines, or EBCPGs. The work of the panel was funded by government and nonprofit organizations in Canada. The purpose of this project was to create clinical guidelines for an aerobic walking program as an intervention to manage osteoarthritis. The panel initially identified more than 700 potential articles. Inclusion and exclusion criteria and a review of each study's methodological quality reduced the number to 7 high-quality studies. Data from studies were combined for a meta-analysis to obtain the results. The panel's conclusion was that an aerobic walking program was an effective short-term intervention for osteoarthritis and provided the greatest improvements in pain, functional level, and quality of life.

As another example, the Orthopedic Section of the American Physical Therapy Association has developed clinical practice guidelines for various orthopedic diagnoses. One of the recently published guidelines presented low back pain guidelines that were linked to the International Classification of Functioning, Disability and Health.[11] The Orthopedic Section appointed content experts to develop the guidelines based on evidence that was available at that time. The panel of experts developed guidelines for diagnosis, examination, and intervention. They recommended a number of interventions that were identified as recommendations based on strong evidence, and those included manual therapy, trunk coordination, strengthening and endurance exercises, directional preference exercises and procedures, and progressive endurance exercise and fitness activities. Interventions based on moderate evidence included patient education and counseling. Interventions supported by weak evidence included flexion exercises and lower quarter nerve mobilization procedures. The panel noted that there was conflicting evidence regarding traction for low back pain.

Learning Task

Using the PEDro website (www. pedro.org.au), locate a clinical practice guideline related to an orthopedic condition that was published within the past 10 years. Read the article and answer the following questions:

• What was the topic of the clinical practice guideline?
• What types of individuals were included in the panel of experts?
• What were the inclusion and exclusion criteria?
• How many studies were initially located? How many were included in the review?
• How many subjects were included in all of the selected studies?
• What was the level of evidence of for each conclusion/recommendation?

Addressing Biases and Threats to Validity

The information provided in this chapter regarding research reviews and clinical guidelines can be helpful to the reader in reviewing and understanding the literature. These types of reviews are a useful tool and can save the clinician time by providing a compilation of multiple studies. Systematic reviews are a key component of evidence based practice. The systematic review can stand alone or form the basis for a meta-analysis or development of clinical guidelines.

We have addressed issues of bias in the previous chapters on research, and bias can be an issue with reviews as well. Let's review the key components of a systematic review and how bias can be addressed. The first component is that the objectives of the review must be clearly outlined and eligibility criteria determined before the review. This will prevent bias by ensuring that the procedures are not influenced by the results of the literature review. The second component is a precise methodology that can be duplicated and updated as needed. This provides transparency in the process and ensures that all studies were addressed in the same manner and using the same guidelines. Another key component of a systematic review is an organized and methodical search that attempts to identify all relevant studies. Why is this important? An exhaustive search can eliminate bias by locating all studies that address a particular topic, not just the ones that are most accessible. A systematic review should typically consist of exhaustive reviews of multiple databases, conference proceedings, review of references of studies identified, and communication with authors for additional information. As noted previously in this textbook, it is more likely that studies with positive findings will be published, which could bias a review that was not exhaustive. Additional components of a systematic review are an appraisal of the validity of the studies' findings and an organized presentation and synthesis of the findings. The authors should be very clear about how the assessment of the studies was conducted and should present an appraisal of each study that met the specified criteria. The authors should also present the synthesis of the findings in an organized format and clearly link the studies' findings with the authors' conclusions.

Meta-analyses and clinical guidelines are based on systematic reviews and should follow the same procedures to ensure that issues with bias are addressed. In addition, studies identified for a meta-analysis must be fairly similar to each other in order for the statistical analysis to be meaningful. For clinical practice guidelines to be used, the panel developing the guidelines should be well qualified and recognized as experts in the area of clinical practice in which the guidelines are being developed.

Application to Evidence Based Practice

Systematic reviews, meta-analyses, and clinical practice guidelines are often identified as key components in evidence based practice. These types of reviews provide a means of consolidating a large amount of evidence into a concise summary that can save a clinician a lot of time in locating evidence. A clinician should be able to identify the type of research review and understand the strengths and limitations of this type of evidence. PTs and PTAs should be able to use research reviews to answer clinical questions and expand their clinical knowledge and expertise. When attempting to answer a clinical question, the clinician will be well served by first searching for systematic reviews or meta-analyses and clinical practice guidelines. If no results are found, the clinician can then move on to the next level of evidence, such as individual experimental research or exploratory research studies.

SUMMARY

This chapter has covered various types of research reviews that are commonly encountered during a review of the literature. Research reviews are considered secondary sources of evidence and include systematic reviews, meta-analyses, and clinical practice guidelines. A systematic review applies the scientific method to a review of the literature. The systematic review will outline methodology and inclusion criteria before the review is initiated in order to reduce bias. Authors of a systematic review will provide an appraisal of each study included in the review and will also provide conclusions and recommendations. A meta-analysis begins with a systematic review, but the results of the studies will be combined and statistically analyzed to improve on the power of a single study. Clinical guidelines will typically include a systematic review and meta-analysis, followed by a number of recommendations made by a panel of experts. Clinical guidelines are designed to provide direction to clinicians for clinical decision-making.

● Case Scenario

You are a PTA living in a rural community and working for a home health agency. You have recently begun working with an 89-year-old woman with a diagnosis of early-stage dementia and multiple falls in recent months. She lives with her daughter and son-in-law, who provide care and assistance as needed. The PT developed a plan of care that included strengthening and balance activities along with education of patient and caregivers. When you arrive for your visit today, the daughter asks you about purchasing hip protectors for her mother because she is very concerned about a fall resulting in a hip fracture. You are not familiar with hip protectors but assure the daughter that you will provide more information on your next visit. When you get back to the office, you conduct a search for hip protectors and find a systematic review that addresses your question. The review included 19 studies, with 14 studies of people in nursing or residential care settings and 5 studies of people living at home. The authors of the systematic review concluded that in older people living in nursing facilities, there is moderate-quality evidence that providing a hip protector probably decreases the risk for hip fracture slightly but may slightly increase the risk for a pelvic fracture. The authors also concluded that in older people living at home, there is moderate-quality evidence that hip protectors have little to no effect on hip fractures.[12]

CASE QUESTIONS

1. How would you proceed with the information you have found?

_____

_____

2. Based on the information provided in the systematic review, do you think the patient's daughter should purchase hip protectors?

_____

_____

3. What other factors should be considered in the decision to purchase hip protectors for this patient?

_____

_____

Review Activities

1. In your own words, briefly explain the differences between a systematic review and a meta-analysis.

   _____

   _____

   _____

   _____

2. What is the purpose of a meta-analysis?

   _____

   _____

   _____

   _____

3. What is the purpose of a clinical practice guideline?

   _____

   _____

   _____

   _____

4. What is the purpose of grading the quality of evidence in a research review?

   _____

   _____

   _____

   _____

MATCHING

_____ 1. Meta-analysis

_____ 2. Clinical practice guideline

_____ 3. Systematic review

_____ 4. Power

_____ 5. Cochrane Collaboration

A. Probability that a study will detect an effect that is statistically significant

B. Evidence based recommendations developed by experts

C. Organization that advocates evidence based decision-making

D. Literature review for a specific question

E. Review that includes statistical analysis of study outcomes

■ References

1. University of Oxford. Centre for Evidence Based Medicine. http://www.cebm.net/. Accessed January 15, 2013.
2. Cochrane Collaboration. The Cochrane Library. http://www.cochrane.org. Accessed July 23, 2015.
3. Adie S, Kwan A, Naylor JM, Harris IA, Mittal R. Cryotherapy following total knee replacement. *Cochrane Database Sys Rev*. 2012;9.
4. Harvey L, Brosseau L, Herbert R. Continuous passive motion following total knee arthroplasty in people with arthritis. *Cochrane Database Sys Rev*. 2014;2.
5. Larmer P, Reay N, Aubert E, Kersten P Systematic review of guidelines for the physical management of osteoarthritis. *Arch Phys Med Rehabil*. 2014;95:375-389.
6. Portney LG, Watkins MP. *Foundations of Clinical Research: Applications to Practice*. Upper Saddle River, NJ: Pearson Education; 2008.
7. Wikipedia. Meta-analysis. www.wikipedia.com. Accessed July 23, 2015.
8. Gill SD, McBurney H. Does exercise reduce pain and improve physical function before hip or knee replacement surgery? A systematic review and meta-analysis of randomized controlled trials. *Arch Phys Med Rehabil*. 2013;94:164-176.
9. Tanaka R, Ozawa J, Kito N, Moriyama H. Efficacy of strengthening or aerobic exercise on pain relief in people with knee osteoarthritis: a systematic review and meta-analysis of randomized controlled trials. *Clin Rehabil*. 2013;27(12):1059-1071.
10. Loew L, Brosseau L, Wells GA, et al. Ottawa Panel evidence-based clinical practice guidelines for aerobic walking programs in the management of osteoarthritis. *Arch Phys Med Rehabil*. 2012;93:1269-1290.
11. Delitto A, George S, Dillen L, et al. Low back pain: clinical practice guidelines linked to the International Classification of Functioning, Disability and Health from the Orthopedic Section of the American Physical Therapy Association. *J Orthop Sports Phys Ther*. 2012;42(4):A1-A57.
12. Santesso N, Carrasco-Labra A, Brignardello-Petersen R. Hip protectors for preventing hip fractures in older people. *Cochrane Database Sys Rev*. 2014;3.

Part Three continues to build on the first two parts of this text and provides greater detail about how to find and utilize evidence. The information provided will assist the reader with developing skills in the evidence based clinical decision-making process. Chapter 9 describes the components of a good clinical question using the acronym PICO—Patients, Interventions, Comparison, and Outcome. The importance of asking the right clinical question will be emphasized because this provides the basis for the literature search. Chapter 10 describes different sources of evidence, such as journals and textbooks. A table of peer-reviewed journals commonly used in physical therapy is provided. The chapter will present a more in-depth discussion of hierarchies of evidence and why some types of evidence are considered stronger than others. Chapter 11 introduces search engines and databases most commonly used in health care, including common library resources and the tools offered through membership in the American Physical Therapy Association. A table of search engines and databases is provided along with a brief description and whether a subscription is required. Chapter 12 introduces commonly used terminology for searches, such as Boolean logic, key words, and MeSH headings. Methods for limiting or broadening a search are explained, and simple methods for tracking search terms and strategies are described. Chapter 13 examines a research article in greater depth. The chapter presents questions that should be considered when critically appraising an article and provides the reader with tools to focus on the most important components of an article. Chapter 14 describes the process of integrating evidence with the clinician's knowledge and the patient's values while working within the plan of care developed by the physical therapist (PT). The overall goal of Part Three is to provide the physical therapist assistant (PTA), as a part of the PT/PTA team, with practical tools for using evidence in the clinical decision-making process.

- Chapter 9: Formulating a Focused Clinical Question
- Chapter 10: Locating the Evidence: Sources and Levels of Evidence
- Chapter 11: Locating the Evidence: Search Engines and Databases
- Chapter 12: Locating the Evidence: Search Strategies
- Chapter 13: Critically Appraising the Evidence
- Chapter 14: Applying the Evidence to Patient Care

Formulating a Focused Clinical Question

Chapter at a Glance

Learning Outcomes

After reading this chapter, the reader will be able to:

· Explain the purpose of a clinical question.
· Describe the difference between a foreground question and a background question.
· Discuss each component of a good clinical question using the PICO format.
· List the types of PICO questions that are commonly used.

Key Terms

· Background question
· Control
· Diagnosis
· Diagnostic test or measure
· Etiology
· Foreground question
· Intervention
· Outcome
· Prognosis

◘ FOOD FOR THOUGHT

You have been working in a skilled nursing facility since you graduated from the PTA program 1 year ago. You have primarily been treating patients with strokes, hip fractures, joint replacements, and cardiopulmonary conditions. You learned during the weekly staffing meeting that a new patient is being admitted who has been diagnosed with amyotrophic lateral sclerosis. You don't know much about this disease, and you want to learn more about the condition.

Questions to consider:
· What clinical question would you ask?
· Would it be a foreground question or a background question?
· What type of resources would you use to find the best information (evidence)?

Introduction

In Chapter 2 we discussed the five steps of the evidence based practice process (Fig. 9.1). This chapter will cover the first step, which is formulating a focused clinical question. A search for evidence begins with a good searchable clinical question. The success of your literature search depends on how well you are able to clearly identify the specifics of the search. A good clinical question will save you time and keep you focused. One commonly used method of developing a clinical question is the acronym PICO (Fig. 9.2). This type of question works particularly well when searching for the answer to a question related to interventions. A search for evidence about diagnosis or prognosis may require a slightly different type of question, but the process for developing the question is essentially the same.

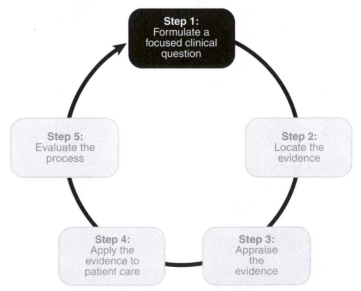

Figure 9.1 The Evidence Based Practice Process is a five-step process. The first step is formulating a focused clinical question.

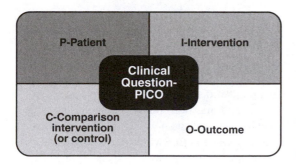

Figure 9.2 The acronym PICO can be used to develop a focused clinical question.

Questions can arise in the clinic at any time, but not all questions will be clinical questions requiring an evidence search (Fig. 9.3). Each patient encounter can give rise to questions such as the following:

- How is the patient doing today compared with the previous visit?
- Has the patient been compliant with the home program?
- If the patient is not progressing as expected, why not? Could another intervention achieve better results?
- How much more can the patient expect to progress?
- Should the intensity of therapy be increased? Decreased?

You may come up with multiple clinical questions during a patient visit, particularly if the patient diagnosis, situation, or response to treatment is unusual. If you come up with more than one clinical question requiring an evidence search, you will need to determine which question is most important at that time or which issue should be addressed first. After you have answered the most important question, you can then follow up with a different question at a later time if needed.

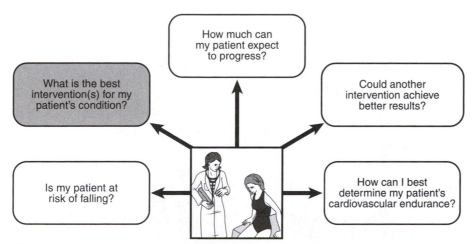

Figure 9.3 Any PTA–patient interaction can lead to questions. However, not all questions will be searchable questions. The PTA must decide which searchable question is most important to be addressed first. In this example, the PTA may decide that the question to be addressed first is "What is the best intervention for my patient's condition?" Source: *Fetters L, Tilson J.* Evidence Based Physical Therapy. *Philadelphia, PA: FA Davis; 2012.*

Types of Questions

Clinical questions can generally be divided into two types of questions: background and foreground. A **background question** focuses on the typical course of a disease or injury or the typical management of a problem.[1-3] Background questions relate to general knowledge about a condition or treatment and are generally broader in scope. New clinicians are likely to have a lot of background questions because they don't yet have the experience needed to develop a broad base of general knowledge. More experienced clinicians will also have background questions when faced with a patient situation that is new or unfamiliar. Specific resources that are helpful for answering background questions include textbooks, professional associations, and national patient advocacy groups. Government agencies may also provide current information for background questions, such as the Centers for Disease Control and Prevention (www.cdc.gov).

A **foreground question** focuses on making clinical decisions related to patient management.[1-3] A foreground question may involve choosing specific tests or interventions for a particular patient or making diagnostic or prognostic decisions. All clinicians should be asking foreground questions on a regular basis because new evidence is continually emerging. The PICO format was primarily developed for answering foreground questions. Specific resources that are helpful in answering foreground questions include professional journals and conference proceedings.

Components of PICO Questions

The first component of a clinical question using the PICO format is P, which can stand for Patient, Population, or Problem, depending on the clinical situation. To make sure your question is focused, you could ask the following questions[4]:

- How could you describe a group with the same or a similar problem?
- How would you describe the patient to another health-care professional?
- What are the key characteristics of your patient and should these be considered when searching for evidence?
  - Primary problem
  - Patient's main concern or chief complaint
  - Disease or health status
  - Age, race, sex, previous ailments, current medications

Consider the following patient scenario:

You are working with a 78-year-old Hispanic woman who has a history of multiple falls in recent months. She was recently hospitalized following a fall from standing height at home with brief loss of consciousness. She was diagnosed with a subdural hematoma of the right temporal lobe.

What key characteristics would be important to include in your question? When developing a searchable question, you should consider that the more specific information you include, the more difficult it will be to find relevant literature. For example, you could write the first part of the question as, "elderly patients with temporal subdural hematoma." You could also write the first part as, "elderly Hispanic female patients with temporal subdural hematoma following a fall from standing height." Do you think you might have greater difficulty finding information relevant to the second question? Which of the key characteristics are critical to your question? A good strategy is to start with fewer key characteristics and conduct your search. If your search produces a large number of results, you can then add more characteristics to narrow your search. For our scenario, we will say: **P** = "elderly patients with temporal subdural hematoma."

The second component of the question is I for Intervention. An **intervention** is a purposeful interaction of a PT or PTA with a patient using physical therapy procedures and techniques to produce change.[5] A clinician who is unfamiliar with common interventions for a particular patient problem might ask a background question. In that instance, the clinician would be looking for a variety of treatment options. However, if the clinician has a specific treatment option in mind for the patient, a foreground question would be more appropriate. Referring back to the patient scenario described previously, let's assume that the patient's primary problem is balance. The clinician might be knowledgeable about balance interventions but unsure which techniques might be best for this patient problem. For our scenario we will say: **I** = "balance activities."

The third component of the question is C for Comparison or Control. A **control** is a designated intervention, or absence of intervention, that will be used as a comparison to the intervention of choice. The control might also be the intervention that is considered the gold standard. This part of the question refers to the control intervention or the comparison intervention and will describe the main alternative to the intervention you are considering. This could be no intervention, a placebo intervention, or the standard treatment. If the clinician is deciding between two alternative interventions, this would be the second intervention being considered. It is not unusual for a clinical question to be written without this component. This is the only component of the question that can be omitted without significantly affecting a searchable clinical question.[6] For our example, we will say: **C** = "no balance activities."

The fourth component of the question is O for Outcome. The **outcome** is the change in condition as a result of the intervention. Describe what would be accomplished, or the outcome that you would like to see for your patient. For this example, we will say: **O** = "dynamic standing balance."

A simple format for writing the PICO question (Table 9.1) for interventions is as follows:

For _____ (P), would _____ (I) compared with _____ (C) affect _____ (O)?

Table 9.1 | Example of an Intervention Question in PICO Format

Question Component	PICO Element	Question
Patient characteristic	P	For elderly patients with temporal subdural hematoma,
Interaction	I	would balance activities
Comparison	C	compared with no balance activities
Outcome	O	affect dynamic standing balance?
	or	
Patient characteristic	P	For elderly patients with temporal subdural hematoma,
Interaction	I	would balance activities
Outcome	O	affect dynamic standing balance?

Our question, after we put all of these components together, would be:

"For elderly patients with temporal subdural hematoma, would balance activities compared with no balance activities **affect** dynamic standing balance?"

We could also write the question to indicate that we want to know if balance activities will improve standing balance rather than just affecting standing balance: "For elderly patients with temporal subdural hematoma, would balance activities compared with no balance activities **improve** dynamic standing balance?"

Learning Task

You are a PTA working in a small community hospital, and the therapist has placed a new patient on your schedule for the following morning. The patient is 85 years old and had surgery 3 days ago for a mitral valve replacement because of mitral valve stenosis. You would like to find evidence about the best types of activities for this patient in the acute care setting to discuss with the therapist before tomorrow's treatment.

Write a PICO question for this scenario.

Using PubMed (www.pubmed.com), search for a research study published within the past 5 years that addresses rehabilitation for patients following mitral valve replacement. Would the study you selected be helpful in answering your clinical question?

Other Types of Foreground Clinical Questions

The discussion so far has focused on foreground clinical questions related specifically to interventions. PTAs will mostly use intervention types of questions because intervention is the primary patient management category for PTAs. However, clinical questions can also address diagnosis or diagnostic tests (i.e., what is the disease or condition?), prognosis (i.e., what is the likely outcome?), or etiology (i.e., what is the cause?). Let's look briefly at each of these types of questions.

Diagnostic Questions

A **diagnosis** is defined as a description of a patient condition derived by evaluating the data obtained during an examination. A **diagnostic test** or **measure** is defined as a measure used to obtain objective information during the diagnostic process.[5] Clinical questions related to diagnosis are generally asking if a specific diagnostic test or measure is accurate. For example, a therapist is working with a patient with a primary diagnosis of chronic obstructive pulmonary disease (COPD). The therapist is considering using the 6-Minute Walk Test with this patient to measure the level of impairment of aerobic capacity and is not sure whether this test is a valid measure in patients with this diagnosis. By slightly altering the original PICO question outline (Table 9.2), a question can be developed related to diagnostics:

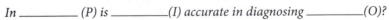

In _____ (P) is _____(I) accurate in diagnosing _____(O)?

A question in this case might be: "In patients with COPD, is the 6-Minute Walk Test accurate in diagnosing impaired aerobic capacity?"

You will notice that the Comparison or Control component of the question was omitted. Why? In this case the therapist did not want to compare the test to another test. The question was whether the test was a valid measure for this type of patient.

Table 9.2 | Example of a Diagnostic Question in PICO Format

Question Component	PICO Element	Question
Patient characteristic	P	In patient with COPD,
Interaction	I	is the 6-Minute Walk Test
Comparison	C	more accurate than the 3-Minute Step Test
Outcome	O	in diagnosing impaired aerobic capacity?
	or	
Patient characteristic	P	In patients with COPD,
Interaction	I	is the 6-Minute Walk Test
Outcome	O	accurate in diagnosing impaired aerobic capacity?

If the therapist wanted to compare two different diagnostic tests, the question could be: "In patients with COPD, is the 6-Minute Walk Test more accurate than the 3-Minute Step Test in diagnosing impaired aerobic capacity?"

Prognosis Questions

Prognosis is defined as the determination of the expected functional outcome and the time frame needed to achieve the outcome.[5] Clinical questions related to prognosis are generally asking if a specific test or measure predicts an outcome. For example, consider that you are treating a 79-year-old woman who is recovering from a femoral neck fracture following open reduction and internal fixation 12 weeks ago. You would like to know whether the Tinetti Performance-Oriented Mobility Assessment (POMA) or the Berg Balance Scale is a better measure for this patient in predicting risk for falling. By again altering the original PICO question outline (Table 9.3), a question can be developed related to prognosis:

> *For _____ (P) how does _____(I) compared to _____(C) predict _____(O)?*

Our question in this case might be: "For elderly females following hip fracture, how does the Tinetti POMA compared with the Berg Balance Scale predict risk for falling?"

A comparison measure is not necessary. A clinician may just want to know if a specific outcome measure predicts an outcome. The question would then be: "For elderly females following hip fracture, does the Tinetti POMA predict risk for falling?"

Etiology Questions

Etiology is defined as the cause of a disease or condition and may include a specific set of factors that contribute to the disease or condition occurrence. Clinical questions related to etiology are generally asking whether a specific factor places a patient at greater risk for a condition. For example, consider that you have just begun treating a 46-year-old man who sustained a tibia/fibula fracture with an open wound. Although the accident occurred several weeks ago, the wound has not completely healed. In reviewing the patient's record, you notice that he smokes two packs of

Table 9.3 | Example of a Prognostic Question in PICO Format

Question Component	PICO Element	Question
Patient characteristic	P	For elderly females following hip fractures,
Interaction	I	how does the Tinetti POMA
Comparison	C	compared with the Berg Balance Scale
Outcome	O	predict risk for falling?
	or	
Patient characteristic	P	For elderly females following hip fractures,
Interaction	I	does the Tinetti POMA
Outcome	O	predict risk for falling?

cigarettes a day. You want to know if significant tobacco use could be a cause of delayed wound healing, and you also would like to know if this could cause delayed bone healing as well. You could use the following format to develop your question (Table 9.4):

Are _____ (P) who _____ (I) compared with those who do not _____(C) at greater risk for _____(O)?

The clinical questions in this case might be: "Are middle-aged males who use tobacco compared with those who do not use tobacco at greater risk for delayed wound healing?"

Or "Are middle-aged males who use tobacco at greater risk for delayed bone healing?"

Foreground clinical questions can be developed to address a wide array of topics, but in each case the basic framework is the PICO format. With practice, clinicians can become skilled at writing focused clinical questions to address a variety of topics.

Table 9.4 | Example of an Etiology Question in PICO Format

Question Component	PICO Element	Question
Patient characteristic	P	Are middle-aged males
Interaction	I	who use tobacco
Comparison	C	compared with nonsmokers
Outcome	O	at greater risk for delayed wound healing?
	or	
Patient characteristic	P	Are middle-aged males
Interaction	I	who use tobacco
Outcome	O	at greater risk for delayed wound healing?

SUMMARY

A focused clinical question is critical to a successful search for evidence. Clinical questions can be classified as background questions or foreground questions. Background questions are typically broad in nature and are used in situations that are unfamiliar to the clinician. Foreground questions are more specific in nature and are used in situations in which the clinician is looking for evidence for specific patient management questions. The acronym PICO (Patient, Intervention, Control, Outcome) is a commonly used method for developing a clinical question. The PICO format is typically used for clinical questions related to interventions. Other types of clinical questions, such as diagnostic, prognostic, or etiology questions, can be addressed using a slight variation of the PICO format.

● Case Scenario

You are working in an outpatient therapy clinic that focuses on the geriatric orthopedic population. The majority of patients treated at the clinic have undergone total joint replacements, such as total knees, total hips, and total shoulders. The therapist that you are teamed with just evaluated a 64-year-old patient who underwent a total ankle replacement 3 weeks ago. The therapist has asked you to place this patient on your schedule for his next appointment. You are not familiar with this type of surgery and want to find out as much about the procedure as possible. You also want to become familiar with exercises that are appropriate for patients following this procedure.

CASE QUESTIONS

1. Write an example of a background question for this scenario.

_____

_____

2. Write an example of a foreground question for this scenario.

_____

_____

3. Which type of question would be most important in preparing to work with this patient?

_____

_____

Learning Task

Using the search tool CINAHL through your library or the American Physical Therapy Association website, conduct a search for a research article about total ankle replacement. Read the article and share the information with your classmates during group discussion.

- Did your article provide information about the procedure itself or about therapy following the procedure?
- Was your article better for answering your background question or your foreground question?
- Did any of the articles provide information about therapeutic interventions, such as exercise?

Review Activities

1. What is the purpose of a clinical question?

_____

_____

_____

_____

2. In your own words, define a foreground question.

_____

_____

_____

_____

3. List two questions that can help a clinician make a clinical question more focused.

_____

_____

_____

_____

4. Which component of the PICO question can be omitted and in what circumstances?

_____

_____

_____

_____

MATCHING

_____ 1. Background question   A. Cause of a disease or condition

_____ 2. Foreground question   B. Change in condition resulting from intervention

_____ 3. Diagnosis   C. Question focused on making clinical decisions

_____ 4. Outcome   D. Description of condition based on examination

_____ 5. Prognosis   E. Question focused on typical course or management of disease

_____ 6. Etiology   F. Expected outcomes and time frame

References

1. Fetters L, Tilson J. *Evidence Based Physical Therapy.* Philadelphia, PA: FA Davis; 2012.
2. Jewell, DV. *Guide to Evidence-Based Physical Therapist Practice.* 3rd ed. Burlington, MA: Jones & Bartlett Learning; 2015.
3. Hack LM, Gwyer J. *Evidence Into Practice: Integrating Judgment, Values and Research.* Philadelphia, PA: FA Davis; 2013.
4. USC website. Evidence Based Decision Making. www.usc.edu/hsc/ebnet/ebframe/PICO.htm#PRef. Accessed July 23, 2015.
5. American Physical Therapy Association (APTA). *Guide to Physical Therapist Practice.* 2nd ed. Alexandria, VA: APTA; 2003.
6. Texas Tech University Health Science Center Libraries. How to Develop a PICO Question. http://www.ttuhsc.edu/libraries/schools/son.aspx. Accessed July 23, 2015.

Chapter 10

Locating the Evidence: Sources and Levels of Evidence

Chapter at a Glance

Learning Outcomes

After reading this chapter, the reader will be able to:

· Describe the differences between filtered and unfiltered sources of evidence.
· Identify commonly used sources of evidence.
· Describe different types of articles found in journals and the purpose of each.
· Discuss the rationale for why some types of evidence are considered stronger than others.

Key Terms

· Case report
· Effect size
· Filtered (secondary) source

· Narrative review
· Peer review
· Research report
· Research review synopsis

· Study synopsis
· Unfiltered (primary) source

▣ FOOD FOR THOUGHT

You are a physical therapist assistant working in an outpatient clinic in a small community. You have been leading an aquatic therapy group session with four elderly patients with knee osteoarthritis. You have been providing education on lifestyle changes that would be of benefit for these patients, including weight loss, exercises to perform at home, and the use of hot or cold packs at home for pain relief. When you arrive to begin the session one day, one of the patients who is fairly new to the group is passing around what appears to be an article highlighting the benefits of a new machine that can be used at home, and the article guarantees improved function and relief of pain or "your money back." She noted the research studies described in the article that proved the machine worked. She told the other patients that she was going to order one and encouraged them to order one as well. She shows the article to you and you immediately notice that it is not actually an article but an advertisement made to look like an article.

Questions to consider:

· Does the patient have a valid piece of evidence?
· How would you address this situation?
· Would it be important to explain about different types of "evidence"?

Introduction

The second step of the evidence based process is locating the evidence (Fig. 10.1). In this chapter, we will discuss different sources and levels of evidence. The clinician must have an understanding of the types of resources that contain evidence in order to locate the best evidence. The clinician must also understand the different levels of evidence in order to locate the least biased and most trustworthy evidence.

Evidence based practice relies on the clinician's ability to find and use evidence. Evidence is defined as the available body of scientific research literature that can be

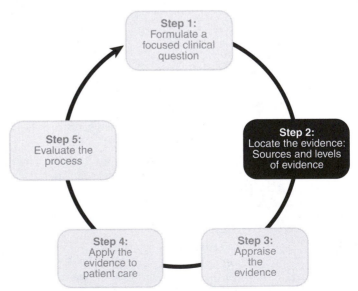

Figure 10.1 The second step of the Evidence Based Practice Process is locating the evidence, which begins with understanding the sources and levels of evidence.

used to answer a clinical question. The past few chapters have provided the reader with information about different types of research that form the foundation of evidence. This chapter will provide an overview of the sources that are commonly used in searching for evidence and will describe the best sources for specific types of evidence. Some types of evidence are considered stronger than others. The chapter will discuss the levels of evidence by reviewing commonly used hierarchies of evidence that rank the types of evidence from strongest to weakest.

Sources of Evidence

In the broadest sense, evidence can be found in a wide range of publications and formats. As a student you likely are using a number of textbooks, which are sources of evidence. You have reviewed journal articles while completing exercises in this text, and these journals and articles are sources of evidence. You may have read an article in a magazine or newspaper describing a new medication or exercise, which would be another source of evidence. Sources of evidence can be categorized as either unfiltered (primary) sources or filtered (secondary) sources. An **unfiltered (primary) source** is defined as a source containing the first report of a study with no outside evaluation or interpretation of the report.[1,2] An example of a primary source would be a research report of a randomized controlled trial (RCT) written by the investigators. A **filtered (secondary) source** is defined as a source that contains information derived from previously published material and includes an evaluation, review, or some other interpretation of the material.[1,2] A filtered source will typically include the author's interpretation and may address more than one research study or report. Following are different types of sources for evidence.

Peer-Reviewed Journals and Articles (Paper, Online)

Professional organizations often publish peer-reviewed journals with the purpose of expanding the body of knowledge within the profession. **Peer review** is defined as the process of evaluation of an article or a similar work by individuals who are considered experts in the field in order to ensure that certain standards are met. Peer-reviewed journals typically include original research reports of the different types of research that were described in Part Two of this text. The *Physical Therapy Journal* (PTJ) is the official journal of the American Physical Therapy Association (APTA) and the Royal Dutch Society for Physical Therapy (KNGF). The *Physical Therapy Journal* was established in 1921 and is the leading physical therapy–specific journal.[3] Several of the APTA sections also publish peer-reviewed journals, including the Sports Medicine, Orthopedic, and Acute Care sections. The journals of other professional associations also serve as excellent resources for physical therapy clinicians. The *Journal of the American Medical Association*, commonly referred to as JAMA, is the official journal of the American Medical Association.[4] Published since 1883, JAMA is the most widely circulated medical journal in the world. Other widely circulated medical journals include the *New England Journal of Medicine* (NEJM) and the *British Medical Journal* (BMJ).[5,6] A number of journals are also geared toward physical medicine and rehabilitation, orthopedics and sports medicine, and allied health. Some nonprofit associations such as the American Heart Association (AHA) also provide peer-reviewed journals. The AHA Scientific Publishing produces several journals, including *Arteriosclerosis, Thrombosis and Vascular Biology* (ATVB), *Stroke*, and *Circulation*.[7] Table 10.1 provides a list of commonly cited journals in physical therapy and rehabilitation literature, but the list is not all-inclusive. Thousands of journals in health care address a wide range of professions, specialties, and topics. Journals have been published on paper for many years, but a number of journals now offer an online option in addition to or instead of a hard copy.

Table 10.1 | Examples of Peer-Reviewed Journals Related to Physical Therapy and Rehabilitation

Peer-Reviewed Journal	Publisher/Sponsor
Physical Therapy	
Physical Therapy Journal (PTJ)	APTA
Journal of Acute Care Physical Therapy (JACPT)	APTA Acute Care Section
Cardiopulmonary Physical Therapy Journal	APTA Cardiovascular and Pulmonary Section
Journal of Physical Therapy Education (JOPTE)	APTA Education Section
Journal of Geriatric Physical Therapy	APTA Geriatrics Section
Physical Therapy Journal of Policy, Administration, and Leadership	APTA Section on Health Policy and Administration
Journal of Neurologic Physical Therapy	APTA Neurology Section
Rehabilitation Oncology	APTA Oncology Section
Journal of Orthopaedic and Sports Physical Therapy (JOSPT)	APTA Orthopedic Section and Sports Medicine Section
Pediatric Physical Therapy	APTA Pediatric Section
International Journal of Sports Physical Therapy (IJSPT)	APTA Sports Medicine Section
Physical Medicine and Rehabilitation	
Archives of Physical Medicine and Rehabilitation	American Congress of Rehabilitation Medicine
Physical Medicine and Rehabilitation Journal	American Academy of Physical Medicine and Rehabilitation
Annals of Physical and Rehabilitation Medicine	French Society of Rehabilitation (SOFMER)
Sports Medicine	
American Journal of Sports Medicine	American Orthopedic Society for Sports Medicine
Medicine and Science in Sports and Exercise	American College of Sports Medicine
Clinical Journal of Sports Medicine	American Medical Society for Sports Medicine
Journal of Athletic Training	National Athletic Trainers Association
Physical Therapy in Sport	Association of Chartered Physiotherapists in Sports and Exercise Medicine
Medicine	
Journal of the American Medical Association (JAMA)	American Medical Association

Table 10.1 | Examples of Peer-Reviewed Journals Related to Physical Therapy and Rehabilitation—cont'd

Peer-Reviewed Journal	Publisher/Sponsor
New England Journal of Medicine (NEJM)	Massachusetts Medical Society
British Medical Journal (BMJ)	British Medical Association
The Lancet	The Lancet/Elsevier
Nursing and Allied Health	
American Journal of Occupational Therapy	American Occupational Therapy Association
American Journal of Nursing	Wolters Kluwer Health/Lippincott
American Journal of Speech-Language Pathology	American Speech-Language-Hearing Association
Journal of the American Association of Nurse Practitioners	American Association of Nurse Practitioners

Peer-reviewed journals, sometimes called scholarly or refereed journals, require authors to submit manuscripts of articles for publication. The manuscripts are reviewed by peers who are considered experts in the field and must meet certain requirements to be reviewers. As an example, the *Journal of Geriatric Physical Therapy* published by the Geriatrics section of the APTA requires manuscript reviewers to have a graduate degree beyond the professional degree (i.e., PhD, EdD) and at least two manuscripts that have been accepted by a peer-reviewed journal.[8] The peer review process may take weeks or months to complete. After an author submits a manuscript, the manuscript is sent to peer reviewers. The reviewers will typically have a designated period of time to complete the initial review. After the review is completed, the editor of the journal will notify the author whether the manuscript has been accepted or rejected. In many instances, the editor will indicate that the manuscript needs to be revised. The author can revise the manuscript and resubmit, at which time the manuscript will be reviewed a second time. At that point, if the revisions meet the expectations of the reviewers and editor, the article will likely be accepted for publication. Some journals are able to publish articles in a short amount of time, whereas other journals may have a long delay between accepting and publishing an article. Many journals now publish an article online fairly quickly after it has been accepted, with a print publication to follow at a later date. Citations for articles will usually indicate when an article was first submitted and when it was accepted for publication. An article about the effectiveness of trigger point dry needling for plantar heel pain was recently published in the *Physical Therapy Journal*.[9] A review of the abstract indicated that the article was originally submitted June 18, 2013 and was accepted March 31, 2014. The article was published online April 3, 2014 and was published in print in the August 2014 issue of the journal.

To determine whether a journal is peer reviewed, a clinician can look at the information on the publishing organization's website or on the information page typically found in the front of the journal. The information may also be found under headings for Authors/Contributors or Reviewers. Journals published by professional organizations are typically peer reviewed. However, certain types of articles published in a peer-reviewed journal may not be peer reviewed, such as editorials or articles from invited authors addressing a specific topic.

Non-Peer-Reviewed Journals and Articles (Paper, Online)

Although many health-care journals are peer reviewed, clinicians may find an article published in a journal that does not require peer review. Journals that are not affiliated with a professional association are less likely to be peer reviewed. Non-peer-reviewed journals accept manuscripts for publication and may require a limited review by an editor or no review at all. Manuscripts are typically published shortly after they are submitted, in contrast to the months-long process normally seen with peer review. Some journals require authors to pay a fee to have their manuscripts published.

One obvious disadvantage of relying on articles from non-peer-reviewed journals is the lack of review by experts knowledgeable about research methodology and about the topic being studied.

Textbooks and Other Educational Materials

Textbooks are written specifically for educational purposes by a single author or multiple authors. Some textbooks have a different authors for each chapter when the textbook covers a large amount of information on a variety of specialized topics. Textbooks may be based on current evidence with many references cited, or based primarily on expert opinion with few references cited. Textbooks provide up-to-date information at the time they are published but may become outdated quickly. Textbooks are frequently updated with newer editions as authors and publishers attempt to incorporate more current information. Other types of educational materials include videos and DVDs, software, and educational websites. Students are familiar with the costs associated with textbooks and educational materials. Many publishers are converting to electronic textbooks, or e-books, to reduce costs of publishing. An advantage of print textbooks is the ability of the clinician to have reference materials readily available in the clinic. A disadvantage of print textbooks is the difficulty with keeping information up to date.

Other Sources

Conference proceedings, or transcripts of professional conferences, are another source of evidence. The transcript may include lectures from invited speakers as well as submitted papers and abstracts. It may also include abstracts of poster or platform presentations from the conference. Government reports and publications are another source of evidence and frequently contain information from recent studies or summaries of research. The Centers for Disease Control and Prevention (www.cdc.gov) and the U.S. Department of Health and Human Services (www.healthfinder.gov) maintain websites with current information on a number of health-related topics (Fig. 10.2).[10,11] Magazines and bulletins are frequently published by professional organizations and may be another source of evidence. The APTA publishes *PT in Motion*, a magazine that highlights news of interest to association members, and *Perspectives*, a magazine for physical therapists (PTs) and physical therapist assistants (PTAs) during the first few years of their career.[3]

An additional source of information is manufacturers' publications, which may include information from studies that present positive outcomes related to their product. They may also provide information from studies that were funded by the manufacturer. The publications may not include research that presented neutral or negative outcomes related to their product and could therefore be biased.[2]

Types of Evidence

In addition to considering the source of the evidence, the reader must also consider the type of evidence. A quick glance at the table of contents of a journal might reveal several research reports, a systematic review or meta-analysis, a case study, and a narrative review (Table 10.2). The most common types of evidence are described next.

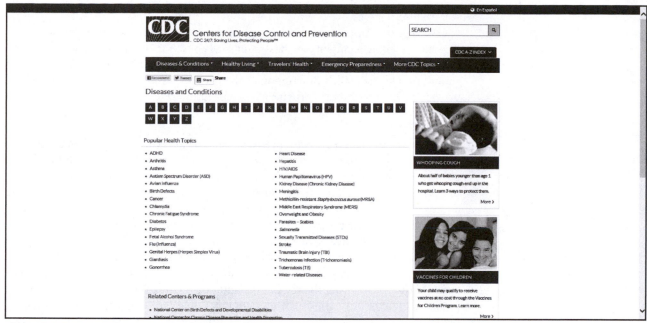

Figure 10.2 Government entities, such as the Centers for Disease Control and Prevention (CDC), maintain websites with current information on a number of health-related topics. *Source:* Screen shot from www.cdc.gov/DiseasesConditions/.

Table 10.2 | Examples of Types of Evidence from March 2015 Physical Therapy Journal*

Type of Evidence	Category in Table of Contents	Title (Author)
Research report	Research reports	"Patients' Use of a Home-Based Virtual Reality System to Provide Rehabilitation of the Upper Limb Following Stroke" (Standen et al.)
Case report	Case reports	"Balance Training Using an iPhone Application in People With Familial Dysautonomia: Three Case Reports" (Gefen et al.)
Narrative review	Perspectives	"Emergence of Virtual Reality as a Tool for Upper Limb Rehabilitation: Incorporation of Motor Control and Motor Learning Principles" (Levin et al.)
Research review	Research reports	"Effectiveness of Passive Physical Modalities for Shoulder Pain: Systematic Review by the Ontario Protocol for Traffic Injury Management Collaboration" (Yu et al.)

*The March 2015 issue of the *Physical Therapy Journal* provided several examples of types of evidence, listed here.

Research Report

A **research report** is a report of original research. A wide range of research types may be addressed in research reports, such as RCTs, cohort studies, case-control studies, normative research, and methodological research. The research report should include a list of authors, an abstract, introduction, description of participants, description of methods, presentation of results, discussion of results, and conclusion. The report should include enough detail to allow another investigator to replicate the study.

Case Report

A **case report** is an in-depth description of a case study or case series. A case report typically describes a patient who has an unusual condition, has an unusual response to conventional treatment, or is undergoing a novel treatment intervention. The report should provide a detailed description of the patients, assessments, and interventions provided. Case reports may provide a basis for future research studies.

Narrative Review

A **narrative review** is a report typically written by an expert in a specified field that provides an overview of a topic. A narrative review includes a discussion of selected articles presented from the author's perspective and is not an exhaustive review of the literature. An invited author's article in a journal covering a topic about which the author is considered an expert is an example of a narrative review. A narrative review addressing home care was published in the *Cleveland Clinic Journal of Medicine* in 2013.[12] The narrative review was written by a physician who was presenting his perspectives about home care following total knee replacement. The physician presented a review of some of the evidence supporting home care following total knee arthroplasty. Throughout the review, the author provided references from previously published studies to support his argument that home care is associated with less cost, better patient outcomes, and greater patient satisfaction. As noted previously, a narrative review presents evidence from the author's viewpoint and is therefore biased. Narrative reviews can be helpful for providing different perspectives on a clinical question or other patient care topic.

Research Reviews

Research reviews, such as systematic reviews and meta-analyses, may be included with research reports in some journals or may be included in a separate section. These types of reports are filtered, or secondary, sources, and provide a critical review and analysis of previously published research. Research reviews include an exhaustive review of the literature with an appraisal of articles based on stringent guidelines. Meta-analyses include a statistical analysis of pooled data from selected studies. Research reviews will include recommendations along with the level of evidence supporting each recommendation.

Clinical Practice Guidelines

Clinical practice guidelines are evidence based recommendations for the diagnosis, treatment, or prevention of health-care problems that are typically developed by a panel of experts. The majority of clinical guidelines are developed through the funding of professional associations, government entities, or health-care organizations. Most clinical practice guidelines will include a systematic review and meta-analysis of the literature followed by recommendations for clinical decision-making. The panel of experts provides clinical expertise in the review of evidence and the development of recommendations. Although similar to a systematic review, clinical practice guidelines are typically broader in scope.

Synopses

A synopsis of evidence can cover individual studies or research reviews. A **study synopsis** is a brief, focused summary of a study that includes commentary by the professional reviewing the study.[13] A synopsis can provide quick advice for busy clinicians because typically only high-quality and clinical relevant articles are selected for a synopsis. The synopsis may appear to be similar to the original abstract of the research article. A key difference, however, is that the abstract is written by the original researcher, whereas the synopsis is written by an expert reviewer. Some journals and websites have been created in recent years with a primary focus of reporting synopses of studies rather than original research. Other journals that primarily report original research have added sections to report synopses of studies. One source of synopses relevant to physical therapy can be found in the American Physical Therapy Association's *Hooked on Evidence*.[14] Information is extracted from research articles and entered into the system by reviewers. Another source of study synopses relevant to therapy is the PEDro database.[15] The organization that developed and maintains this database, the Centre for Evidence Based Physiotherapy, also developed the PEDro scale for assessing the quality of a study. All RCTs listed in the PEDro database are rated, and the PEDro score is listed along with the name of the article.

A **research review synopsis** is a brief, focused summary of a systematic review or meta-analysis that includes commentary by the professional completing the synopsis.[13] Systematic reviews and meta-analyses, which by definition include a comprehensive review of a topic, can be very lengthy and difficult to read. A synopsis of a research review will provide a quick summary of the review's results and will typically address the reliability of the authors' conclusions. The Database of Abstracts of Reviews of Effects (DARE) is the largest source of this type of synopsis.[16] Just as a systematic review or meta-analysis can save the clinician time by consolidating a lot of information, the synopsis can provide a very quick summary of a large amount of information.

Levels of Evidence

With a multitude of sources available, how can you determine whether a source of evidence is trustworthy? A clinician expects to be able to trust that evidence is accurate and has been reviewed in an objective and nonbiased manner. Peer-reviewed journals are typically considered the most trustworthy, particularly journals that use a blinded peer review process.[4] A blinded review process means that experts assigned to review a manuscript are not provided with the author's name. The blinded process should prevent a positive or negative bias in the review because of name recognition of the manuscript author. In addition, journals typically require authors to identify conflicts of interest, such as funding sources that might appear to present the potential for bias. Manufacturers' claims are typically considered the least trustworthy because the line between evidence and product promotion may not be clear. The motivation of the authors and publishers should be considered when trying to determine trustworthiness.

When a clinician is searching for evidence related to a clinical question, the clinician must understand the strength and quality of the evidence. As an example, assume that you have located three articles relevant to your clinical question: a report of an original research study, a systematic review, and a report of a case study. Would all three articles be useful to you? Which one would be considered the strongest evidence? Which would be considered the weakest evidence? Several different hierarchies of evidence showing strongest to weakest can be found in the literature, but none is universally accepted. The levels of evidence will vary to some extent depending on the purpose of the research: intervention, diagnosis, or prognosis.

Figure 10.3 depicts a hierarchy of evidence that was presented earlier in the text. In this hierarchy, expert opinion, editorials, and narrative reviews are some of the weakest types of evidence because they are subjective and based on an individual's opinion or perception. Case reports and case series are examples of descriptive research and represent slightly stronger evidence. Exploratory research, such as case-control studies and cohort studies, represents stronger evidence than description research or opinion because it includes the collection and analysis of data following stringent guidelines. RCTs are stronger than other types of research because they

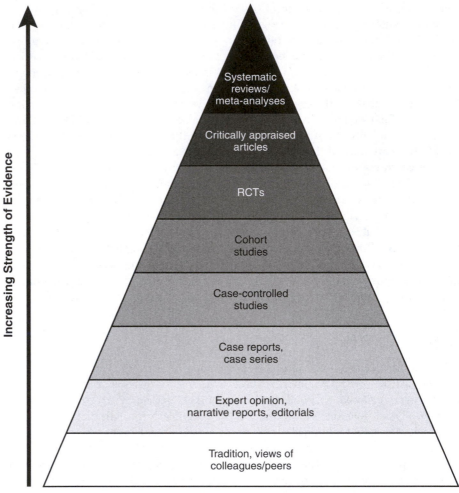

Figure 10.3 A hierarchy of evidence for clinical decision-making depicts the strength of different sources of evidence. The higher levels on the pyramid represent stronger evidence. RCTs, randomized controlled trials.

are the most rigorous type of study. Critically appraised articles and research reviews are the strongest type of evidence in this hierarchy because they include critical appraisal of the original research.

Grading and Quality of Evidence

Research reviews typically incorporate some type of grading system to assess the quality of the evidence. Some grading systems will include four categories of quality: high, moderate, low, and very low.[17] Other grading systems may include fewer categories. Regardless of the grading system, an RCT will generally be rated as high-quality evidence, whereas exploratory and observational studies will generally be rated as low-quality evidence. A thorough review of each study can result in the initial grade being lowered or raised. For example, an RCT would start as high quality, but the grade could be lowered depending on the reviewer's assessment of limitations in the study's design, variability in the study's results, or small effect size. An observational study would start as low quality, but the grade could be raised if the study showed a large effect size. An **effect size** is defined as the quantitative expression of the magnitude of the difference between two groups or the magnitude of the relationship between two variables.[13] An article written by the GRADE (Grading of Recommendations, Assessment, Development, and Evaluation) Working Group suggested that high-quality evidence should be evidence that would likely not be affected by further research. In other words, the authors are confident that the estimates of effect are accurate. Very-low-quality evidence would include evidence about which any estimate of effect would be very uncertain.[18]

The PEDro Rating Scale is commonly used in physical therapy research reviews. PEDro is a free physical therapy database maintained by the University of Sydney in Australia.[15] The PEDro scale was developed in 1998 to assist users of the PEDro database to quickly determine the quality of studies cited in the database. The scale addresses a number of items related to a study's quality, such as blinding, random assignment, identification of eligibility criteria, and reported results. Using the PEDro scale, each study will be assigned a grade on a scale of 0 to 10 (Table 10.3). Authors should identify the cutoff score that was used to consider a study as high quality (i.e., 7/10).

Learning Task

Go to the PEDro website (www. pedro.org.au) and locate the PEDro Rating Scale under Downloads. Review the criteria that are used to rate RCTs. Next, conduct a simple search for an RCT on any topic. From your search results, find three RCTs that have been rated and review the reasons for the ratings.

• What were the main strengths that contributed in the ratings?
• What were the main deficiencies that contributed to the ratings?

Learning Task

Using PubMed (www.pubmed.com), locate a clinical practice guideline related to physical therapy. Locate the rating scale or scales that were used by the authors and answer the following questions:

• Did the authors rate each individual study selected for review?
• If so, what were the rating criteria for the individual studies?
• Did the authors assign a rating or grade for the supporting evidence of each recommendation?
• If so, what were the rating criteria for the recommendations?
• Discuss with your classmates the purpose of the rating grading scales. In your opinion, would it be helpful if there were one universally recognized rating system for evidence?

Table 10.3 | Examples of Items From the PEDro Scale*

Element	Item on PEDro Scale
Eligibility criteria	Eligibility criteria were specified.
Random assignment	Subjects were randomly allocated to groups.
Blinding	There was blinding of all subjects.
	There was blinding of all therapists who administered the therapy.
	There was blinding of all assessors who measured at least one key outcome.

*The PEDro scale is available at http://www.pedro.org.au/wp-content/uploads/PEDro_scale.pdf.

SUMMARY

This chapter has provided an overview of sources of evidence, types of evidence, and levels of evidence. A variety of sources of evidence exist, including peer-reviewed journals, non-peer-reviewed journals, textbooks, conference proceedings, government reports and publications, magazines and bulletins, and manufacturers' publications. Types of evidence include research reports, case reports, narrative reviews, systematic reviews, meta-analyses, clinical practice guidelines, synopses of studies, and synopses of research reviews. Levels of evidence are related to the quality and strength of the evidence. The clinician needs to understand how levels of evidence are determined to ensure that the strongest available evidence is used in making clinical decisions.

● Case Scenario

You have recently begun working in a 20-bed inpatient rehabilitation unit in a small regional hospital. The unit recently admitted a patient who was involved in a motorcycle crash and sustained a brain injury. The therapist evaluated the patient and determined that he is a level 4 on the Rancho Los Amigos Scale. He is exhibiting aggressive behaviors, difficulty focusing on tasks, and restless wandering behavior. You have been assisting the therapist with treatments for the past few days because it requires two clinicians to assist with balance and safety while helping the patient to attempt certain tasks. The therapist will be out of town for a few days and has asked you to work with another PT while she is out. She has asked you to bring her some ideas and suggestions for treatment, focusing on reducing agitation and facilitating calm behavior. She wants to discuss the ideas and suggestions before she leaves to ensure that the patient's treatment continues as planned.

CASE QUESTIONS

1. What would be your first step in searching for new information?

_____

_____

2. Would you rely on one source for evidence or would you use multiple sources?

_____

_____

3. Find a piece of evidence that would fulfill the therapist's request for information.

_____

_____

Review Activities

1. Describe the difference between filtered and unfiltered sources of information.

   _____

   _____

   _____

   _____

2. Explain the importance of peer review in the publication of journal articles.

   _____

   _____

   _____

   _____

3. Identify four commonly used sources of evidence.

   _____

   _____

   _____

   _____

4. Compare and contrast a research report and a narrative review.

   _____

   _____

   _____

   _____

5. Summarize why the hierarchy of evidence is important to clinicians searching for evidence.

   _____

   _____

   _____

   _____

MATCHING

_____ 1. Primary source   A. An expert overview of a topic

_____ 2. Secondary source   B. Source containing first report of a study

_____ 3. Research report   C. Description of individual patient management

_____ 4. Case report   D. Source that includes report of a study with an appraisal

_____ 5. Narrative review   E. Brief, focused summary with commentary

_____ 6. Study synopsis   F. Report of an original investigation

References

1. Evidence-Based Behavioral-Practice Project. Searching for evidence. http://www.ebbp.org/course_outlines/searching_for_evidence. Accessed July 24, 2015.
2. Helewa A, Walker JM. *Critical Evaluation of Research in Physical Rehabilitation.* Philadelphia, PA: Saunders; 2000.
3. American Physical Therapy Association. APTA website. www.apta.org. Accessed July 24, 2015.
4. American Medical Association. AMA website. www.ama-assn.org. Accessed July 24, 2015.
5. *New England Journal of Medicine.* NEJM website. www.nejm.org. Accessed July 24, 2015.
6. *British Medical Journal.* BMJ website. www.bmj.com/thebmj. Accessed July 24, 2015.
7. American Heart Association. AHA website. http://my.americanheart.org. Accessed July 24, 2015.
8. Section on Geriatrics of American Physical Therapy Association. *Journal of Geriatric Physical Therapy.* http://journals.lww.com/jgpt/pages/default.aspx. Accessed July 24, 2015.
9. Cotchett MP, Munteanu SE, Landorf KB. Effectiveness of trigger point dry needling for plantar heel pain: a randomized controlled trial. *Phys Ther.* 2014;94(8):1083-1094.
10. Centers for Disease Control and Prevention. CDC website. www.cdc.gov. Accessed July 24, 2015.
11. U.S. Department of Health and Human Services. HealthFinder website. www.healthfinder.gov. Accessed July 24, 2015.
12. Froimson MI. In-home care following total knee replacement. *Cleve Clin J Med.* 2013;80:eS15-18.
13. Hack LM, Gwyer J. *Evidence Into Practice: Integrating Judgment, Values, and Research.* Philadelphia, PA: FA Davis; 2013.
14. American Physical Therapy Association. *Hooked on Evidence* database website. http://www.hookedonevidence.com/captcha.cfm. Accessed July 24, 2015.
15. Centre for Evidence Based Physiotherapy. PEDro website. www.pedro.org.au. Accessed July 24, 2015.
16. University of York Centre for Reviews and Dissemination. DARE website. www.crd.york.ac.uk/CRDWEb/. Accessed July 24, 2015.
17. Guyatt GH, Oxman AD, Vist GE, Kunz R, Falck-Ytter Y, Schunemann HJ. GRADE: what is "Quality of Evidence" and why is it important to clinicians. *BMJ.* 2008;336;995-998.
18. GRADE Working Group. Grading quality of evidence and strength of recommendations. *BMJ.* 2004;328:1490-1494.

Locating the Evidence: Search Engines and Databases

Chapter at a Glance

Learning Outcomes

After reading this chapter, the reader will be able to:

· Identify search engines and databases that are relevant to health care and physical therapy.
· Describe the difference between a search engine and a database.
· Identify the main focus of selected databases and search engines.
· Explain the benefit of being a member of a professional association such as the American Physical Therapy Association (APTA) in terms of searching for evidence.

Key Terms

· CINAHL
· Cochrane Library
· DARE
· MEDLINE
· PEDro
· PTNow
· SPORTDiscus

◘ FOOD FOR THOUGHT

You are a physical therapist assistant working in a pediatric clinic. During lunch, you and your supervising therapist were discussing a couple of patients on your caseload who both have a diagnosis of idiopathic toe walking. You have tried several different treatment strategies to address the gait pattern, but the gait is not improving. The therapist suggests that you search the literature for current evidence related to idiopathic toe walking. Your clinic does not have access to a medical library, but you have access to the Internet in the clinic office.

Questions to consider:
· Do you think you would be able to conduct a search for evidence without access to any specialized search tools?
· Do you think you would have more or less difficulty finding articles than you would in a medical library?
· Would being a member of the APTA be of any benefit?

Introduction

In Chapter 10, we discussed different sources and levels of evidence in order to begin locating evidence. In this chapter, we will continue with the second step of the evidence based practice process (Fig. 11.1) by learning to select the most appropriate search tools. A large number of tools are available for conducting a search of the literature online, and this can often lead to confusion about which tool may be best for a particular search. Clinicians should be familiar with the basics of the most commonly used search engines and databases that are relevant to physical therapy.

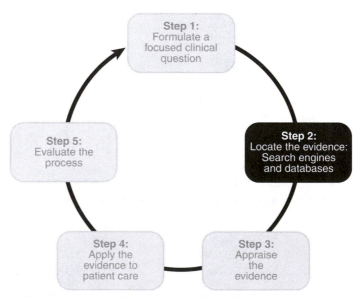

Figure 11.1 The second step of the Evidence Based Practice Process is locating the evidence. The clinician should be familiar with the most common search engines and databases related to physical therapy in order to locate the best evidence.

A search engine is defined as "an information retrieval system that searches the Internet and electronic databases for websites, files or documents based on keywords or phrases."[1] Some search engines, called meta-search engines, are able to search multiple search engines and databases at the same time. Using a meta-search engine can be an efficient means of searching a wide array of resources in a single search. Examples of search engines include the American Physical Therapy Association (APTA) Article-Search, PubMed, and Google Scholar (Figs. 11.2 and 11.3). A *database* is defined as an organized system or collection of citations that allow search access to locate references.[2] Some databases contain primarily citations or abstracts of journal articles and references, whereas other databases also include the full text of articles. Examples of databases include the Cochrane Database of Systematic Reviews, MEDLINE, and PEDro. The reader should keep in mind that electronic search engines and databases range from very broad to very specific in relation to discipline or aspect of patient management. Some focus on filtered resources, whereas others primarily consist of unfiltered original works. Table 11.1 provides a list of commonly used search engines and databases for health sciences that might be useful to physical therapy clinicians. Keep in mind that this list is not all-inclusive, so clinicians may find other search tools that are useful as well.

Most searches of the literature are conducted electronically, but some searches can also be conducted using print sources. Librarians or information technology experts can be very helpful in conducting a search, so don't be afraid to ask questions. Information technology strategies in recent years have led to advances in the synthesis and organization of research evidence.[1] These advances can provide much quicker access to the evidence than in years past. A few of the most commonly used search engines and databases from Table 11.1 are outlined here. The focus area of each search tool is

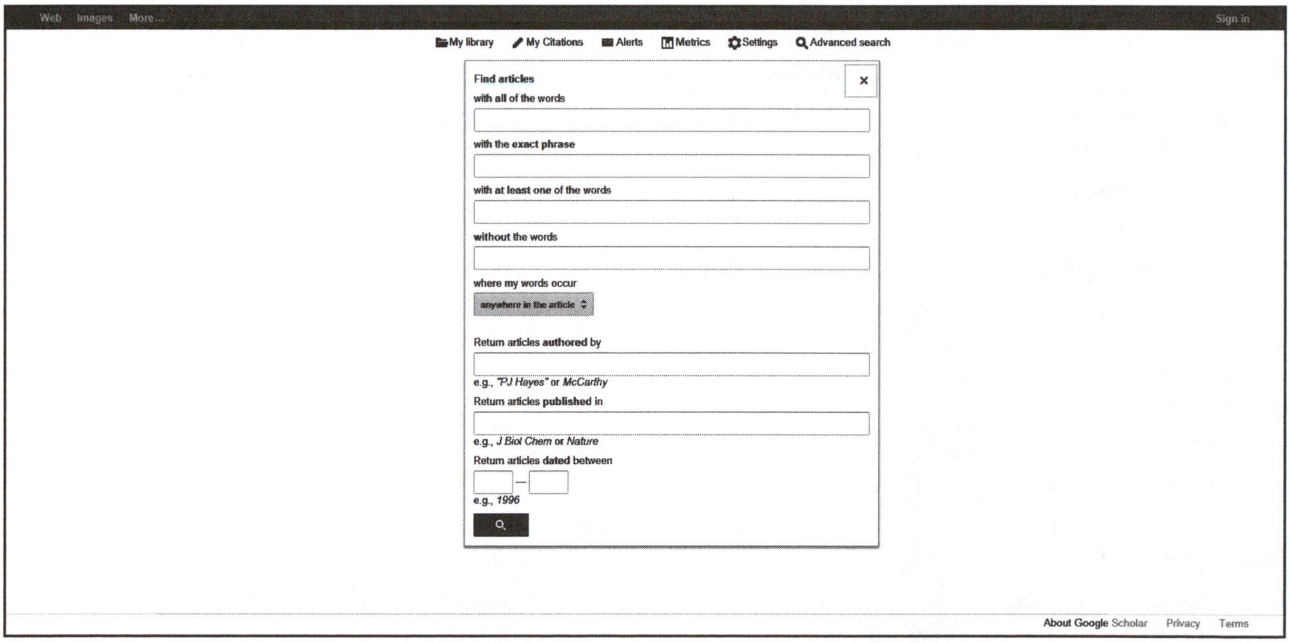

Figure 11.2 Google Scholar is a publicly available search engine, and it includes an advanced search option (see screenshot). The advanced search option allows the user to search by key words or phrases, by author, by journal, and by publication dates. Google Scholar is available at http://scholar.google.com/.

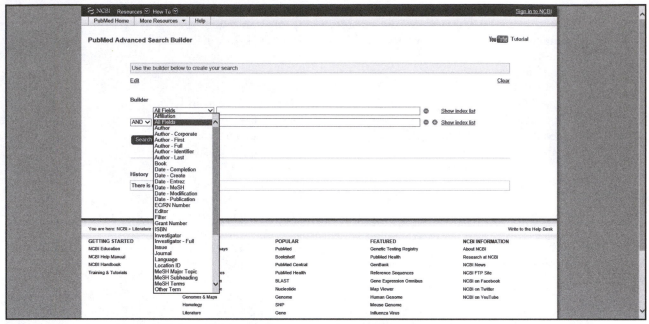

Figure 11.3 PubMed is a publicly available search engine with an advanced search option (see screenshot). The advanced search option allows the user to search using a number of options from drop-down menus. PubMed is available at http://www.ncbi.nlm.nih.gov/pubmed.

Table 11.1 | Commonly Used Bibliographic Search Engines and Databases Related to Health Care

Source	Website	Focus	Requires Subscription
CINAHL: Cumulative Index of Nursing and Allied Health Literature	www.cinahl.com	Nursing, allied health	Yes
BMJ Clinical Evidence	www.clinicalevidence.com	Systematic reviews, medicine	Yes
Clinical Trials Registry	www.clinicaltrials.gov	Summaries of clinical trials and interventional studies	No
Cochrane Collaboration (Cochrane Library)	www.cochrane.org	Systematic reviews, clinical trials	No
DARE: Database of Abstracts of Reviews of Effects	www.york.ac.uk/inst/crd	Abstracts of systematic reviews of interventions	No
Evidence Based Decision Making Journal Club	www.evidencebased.net	Critically appraised health-care articles	No
Evidence-Based Practice Centers (EPC) Reports	www.ahrq.gov/clinic/epc	Reports on evidence based practice topics	No
Google Scholar	www.scholar.google.com	None	No
MEDLINE/PubMed	www.pubmed.gov	Medical, health care	No

Table 11.1 | Commonly Used Bibliographic Search Engines and Databases Related to Health Care—cont'd

Source	Website	Focus	Requires Subscription
National Guideline Clearinghouse	www.guideline.gov	Clinical practice guidelines	No
National Rehabilitation Information Center (NARIC)	www.naric.com	Rehabilitation	No
OTSeeker: OT Systematic Evaluation of Evidence	www.otseeker.com	Systematic reviews, randomized controlled trials	No
PEDro: Physiotherapy Evidence Database	www.pedro.org.au	Physical therapy	No
ProQuest Dissertations and Theses	www.proquest.com	Graduate scholarly products	Yes
ProQuest Nursing and Allied Health Source	www.proquest.com	Nursing, other health professions	Yes
ProQuest Health and Medical Complete	www.proquest.com	Medicine, health care	Yes
PTNow	www.ptnow.org	Physical therapy, allied health	Yes
Public Library of Science (PLoS)	www.plos.org	Medicine, science	No
Rehab+	http://plus.mcmaster.ca/Rehab/Default.aspx	Critically appraised citations	Yes
Scopus	www.scopus.com	Scientific, technical, medical, and social sciences	Yes
SportDiscus	www.ebscohost.com	Sports medicine	Yes
The Dome	www.asha.org	Speech pathology	Yes

also described. The following are provided in alphabetical order, and sites that require a subscription are designated with an asterisk (*).

*CINAHL: Cumulative Index to Nursing and Allied Health Literature

The Cumulative Index to Nursing and Allied Health Literature, or **CINAHL** (www.cinahl.com), is a database that indexes more than 5,000 journals from nursing and other health-care disciplines, including physical therapy.[3] Full-text articles are available from more than 1,300 journals. The *Physical Therapy Journal* is indexed in CINAHL, as well as the journals of a number of APTA sections, such as Acute Care, Geriatrics, Orthopedic/Sports, and Neurologic. The CINAHL database requires a subscription. Students can typically access this database through the school library, and clinicians and students can access CINAHL as APTA members through the APTA website.

*Cochrane Database of Systematic Reviews

The Cochrane Database of Systematic Reviews (www.cochrane.org) is a database that produces and indexes health- and health-care-related systematic reviews and other synthesized research evidence.[4] This database is maintained by the Cochrane Collaboration within the **Cochrane Library** (Fig. 11.4). The Cochrane databases require a subscription. Students may be able to access this database through the school library, and clinicians and students can access Cochrane databases as APTA members through the APTA website.

DARE: Database of Abstracts of Reviews of Effects

The Database of Abstracts of Reviews of Effects (DARE) is one of four databases developed by the Centre for Reviews and Dissemination, University of York (United Kingdom).[5] The **DARE** database (www.york.ac.uk/inst/crd) focuses primarily on systematic reviews of the effects of health-care interventions. The database also includes records of Cochrane reviews and protocols. Critical commentary is added to the reviews by researchers who are knowledgeable about systematic review methods. This commentary can be helpful to the clinician in determining the quality of the review. DARE does not require a subscription.

Google Scholar

Google Scholar (www.googlescholar.com) is a search engine that searches a variety of sources, including journal articles, theses, books, abstracts, and court opinions.[6] Google Scholar indexes individual articles rather than journals and searches a wider variety of sources than other search tools that are geared toward a specific discipline. As a result, a search in Google Scholar will typically provide a much larger number of results. Abstracts and some full-text articles are provided free of charge, but many abstracts will link to a source that is not free. Students and clinicians might need to access another search tool or database to obtain the articles. Google Scholar may be a good tool for a preliminary comprehensive search.

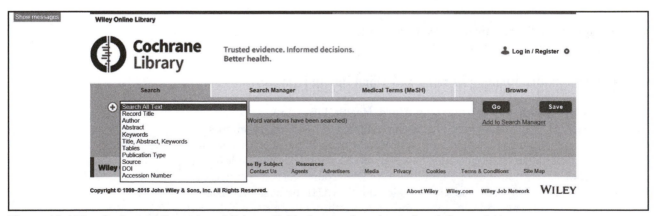

Figure 11.4 The Cochrane Library is publicly available (screenshot shown here) for retrieving abstracts but requires a subscription to retrieve articles. The Cochrane Library is available at http://www.cochranelibrary.com/.

MEDLINE/PubMed

MEDLINE (www.pubmed.gov) is a biomedical database maintained by the National Library of Medicine, which is the world's largest biomedical library.[7] MEDLINE is the most commonly used database in health-related sciences. This database indexes more than 5,600 journals from across the world, with more than 21 million references. MEDLINE can be accessed without a subscription through PubMed and can also be accessed through many institutional libraries. PubMed also includes free access to full-text articles that are archived in PubMed Central, which is a digital archive for articles that are deposited by journals directly into the archive.

National Guideline Clearinghouse

The National Guideline Clearinghouse (NGC) (www.guideline.gov) is a database of clinical practice guidelines maintained by the Agency for Healthcare Research and Quality (AHRQ), which is part of the U.S. Department of Health and Human Services.[8] The clinical practice guidelines that are included in the database are standardized and must meet specific guidelines to be included. NGC does not require a subscription, so it is fully accessible to students and clinicians (Fig. 11.5).

PEDro: Physiotherapy Evidence Database

The Physiotherapy Evidence Database, or **PEDro** (www.pedro.org.au), is a database of more than 27,000 abstracts of clinical trials, systematic reviews, and clinical practice guidelines related to physical therapy (Fig. 11.6).[9] The database is produced by the Centre for Evidence Based Physiotherapy of the George Institute for Global Health, University of

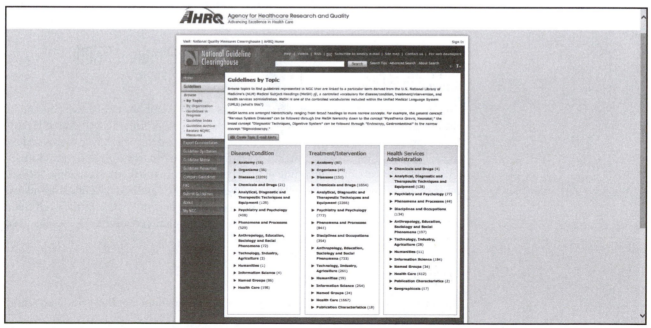

Figure 11.5 The National Guideline Clearinghouse is publicly available (screenshot shown here) for locating clinical practice guidelines in health care. The National Guideline Clearinghouse can be accessed at http://www.guideline.gov/.

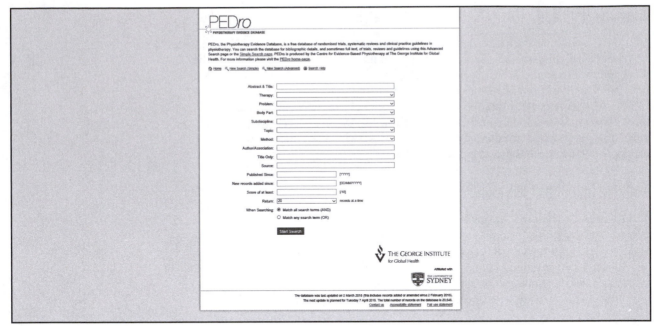

Figure 11.6 The Physiotherapy Evidence Database, or PEDro (see screenshot), is publicly available and contains abstracts of clinical trials, systematic reviews, and clinical practice guidelines related to physical therapy. PEDro can be accessed at http://www.pedro.org.au/.

Sydney (Australia). A standardized rating scale, called the PEDro scale, is used for all clinical trials to assess methodological quality. This rating may be helpful to clinicians, particularly those who are inexperienced at appraising the quality of articles. PEDro does not require a subscription and can be readily accessed by students and clinicians.

*ProQuest Nursing and Allied Health Source and ProQuest Health and Medical Complete

ProQuest is a private company that maintains a large number of databases, and all of the databases require a subscription.[10] Both the ProQuest Nursing and Allied Health Source and the ProQuest Health and Medical Complete databases cover topics related to health care. The nursing and allied health database focuses on nursing and other allied health professions (including physical therapy), and the medical database focuses more on medicine and articles related to physicians. The databases also include videos, e-books, and dissertations. Students may be able to access ProQuest through their institution's library. Clinicians and students who are members of the APTA also have access to ProQuest as a benefit of membership.

*ProQuest Dissertations and Theses

ProQuest Dissertations and Theses is a database of more than 2 million graduate scholarly products.[10] Most of the theses and dissertations are available as full-text items. This database provides access to resources that may not be available through other search engines or databases. As with other ProQuest resources, a subscription is required. This database can be accessed through university libraries or through the APTA.

*PTNow

PTNow (www.ptnow.org) is the research tool for members of the APTA and is available only to members of the association.[11] The tool is made up of several different components. One section, titled Clinical Summaries, consists of summaries that "synthesize evidence-based information about classification, screening, examination, diagnosis, prognosis, and intervention for specific conditions in specific patient populations."[11] The summaries are written by clinicians and are peer reviewed. Clinical Summaries are designed to be concise summaries that provide critical information for clinicians about a particular topic. Another section, titled Guidelines, provides links to clinical practice guidelines that are relevant to physical therapy. The clinical practice guidelines follow the inclusion guidelines of the National Guideline Clearinghouse and have all been published within the previous 5 years.

The primary tool for conducting a literature search on PTNow is a search engine called ArticleSearch (previously called Open Door). ArticleSearch encompasses 10 databases, including Cochrane, ProQuest, SPORTDiscus, DARE, and CINAHL, so it is an efficient search tool. Students and clinicians must be members of the APTA to access ArticleSearch. PTNow also includes other resources, such as Clinical Case reports that illustrate a Clinical Summary, and a large database of Tests and Measures.

*SPORTDiscus

SPORTDiscus is a comprehensive database produced by EBSCO Publishing that is focused on sports and sports medicine.[12] The database provides access to full-text articles from more than 530 journals as well as books, book chapters, and conference proceedings. Subject areas include kinesiology, physical therapy, sports medicine, sports psychology, and physical fitness. SPORTDiscus requires a subscription, so students and clinicians will need to access the database through their institution's library or as members of the APTA.

Additional search engines and databases are listed in Table 11.1, and the reader is encouraged to visit the websites and practice searching on a variety of these sites. These descriptions may seem somewhat confusing because many of these search tools include other search engines and databases in their searches. For example, assume that you want to conduct a search using CINAHL because CINAHL indexes the *Physical Therapy Journal* and a number of other therapy journals. How could you access CINAHL? Figure 11.7 outlines several options for accessing a CINAHL search. A student can go to the school library, and if the school library subscribes to CINAHL, the student can log in and access it. Most colleges and universities that have health-care programs subscribe to CINAHL. A clinician who is practicing at a large medical center may have access through the medical center's library. If neither of these options is available, a student or clinician who is a member of the APTA can access CINHL through the APTA website using ArticleSearch. The ability to access a number of search tools is one benefit of membership in the APTA. Most professional associations offer similar benefits to facilitate evidence based practice.

Learning Task

Select one search tool from Table 11.1 that was not discussed in the chapter. Go to the website listed and find out as much information as you can about the database or search engine, such as:

• Supporting organization
• Specific focus, including health-care professions, types of articles, and so forth
• Number of journals and articles that can be accessed

  Share your findings with your classmates.

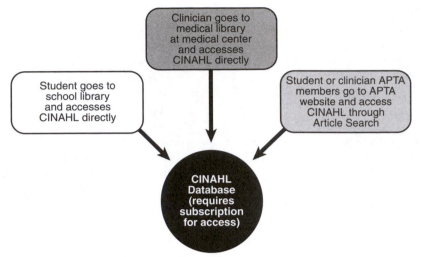

Figure 11.7 Students and clinicians can access a search engine or database in a variety of ways. In this example, CINAHL, which requires a subscription, can be accessed by students and clinicians in more than one way.

SUMMARY

This chapter provided an overview of search engines and databases relevant to physical therapy. A search engine is a retrieval system that searches the Internet based on keywords, whereas a database is a collection of citations that can be searched to access articles and other sources of evidence. A number of search engines and databases require a subscription in order for the user to access them. These include CINAHL, Cochrane, ProQuest, PTNow, and SPORTDiscus. Other search engines and databases are free to the user and can be accessed through most Internet connections. These include DARE, Google Scholar, MEDLINE/PubMed, National Guideline Clearinghouse, and PEDro. Table 11.1 provides a more comprehensive list of search tools available to clinicians for searching the literature.

● Case Scenario

Let's go back to the scenario at the beginning of the chapter. You are a physical therapist assistant working in a pediatric clinic. During lunch, you and your supervising therapist were discussing a couple of patients on your caseload who both have a diagnosis of idiopathic toe walking. You have tried several different treatment strategies to address the limitations, but the gait is not improving. The therapist suggests that you search the literature to see if you can find clinical practice guidelines related to idiopathic toe walking. Your clinic does not have access to a medical library, but you have access to the Internet in the clinic office.

CASE QUESTIONS

1. Which of the search engines or databases would you choose to use? List the top three options.

_____

_____

2. What would be the advantage of locating a clinical practice guideline versus finding an intervention study?

_____

_____

3. If you were able to locate a clinical practice guideline, would you need to discuss the guidelines with the therapist before implementing the recommendations?

_____

_____

Learning Task

Using your top selection of search tools above, locate a clinical practice guideline that addresses this clinical scenario. If you can't locate a clinical practice guideline, locate another type of research article. Read the article and share with your classmates during group discussion.

Review Activities

1. Briefly explain the difference between a search engine and a database.

   _____

   _____

   _____

   _____

2. List three search engines or databases that require a subscription and identify the primary focus of each.

   _____

   _____

   _____

   _____

3. Identify two ways that a student may be able to access databases that require a subscription.

   _____

   _____

   _____

   _____

4. Identify three search engines or databases that do not require a subscription and identify the primary focus of each.

   _____

   _____

   _____

   _____

5. From Table 11.1, identify a search tool that focuses on:

   a. Systematic reviews _____

   b. Clinical practice guidelines _____

   c. Graduate scholarly products _____

MATCHING

_____ 1. PEDro	A. Research tool for APTA members
_____ 2. SPORTDiscus	B. Database for nursing and allied health journals
_____ 3. CINAHL	C. Database of abstracts related to physical therapy
_____ 4. MEDLINE	D. Database maintained by National Library of Medicine
_____ 5. PTNow	E. Database of systematic reviews of health care interventions
_____ 6. DARE	F. Database for sports medicine journals

■ References

1. Portney L, Watkins MP. *Foundations of Clinical Research: Applications to Practice.* Upper Saddle River, NJ: Pearson Education; 2009.
2. Helewa A, Walker JM. *Critical Evaluation of Research in Physical Rehabilitation: Towards Evidence-Based Practice.* Philadelphia, PA: Saunders; 2000.
3. EBSCOhost. Cumulative Index to Nursing and Allied Health. www.ebscohost.com. Accessed July 24, 2015.
4. Cochrane Collaboration. The Cochrane Library. www.cochrane.org. Accessed July 24, 2015.
5. Centre for Reviews and Dissemination, University of York. Database of Abstracts of Reviews of Effects. www.york.ac.uk/inst/crd. Accessed July 24, 2015.
6. Google Scholar. About Google Scholar. http://scholar.google.com/intl/en/scholar/about.html. Accessed July 24, 2015.
7. National Library of Medicine. Fact sheet: MEDLINE. http://www.nlm.nih.gov/pubs/factsheets/medline.html. Accessed July 24, 2015.
8. Agency for Healthcare Research and Quality. National Guideline Clearinghouse. http://www.guideline.gov. Accessed July 24, 2015.
9. Centre for Evidence Based Physiotherapy, University of Sydney. Physiotherapy Evidence Database. http://www.pedro.org.au. Accessed July 24, 2015.
10. ProQuest. ProQuest list of databases. www.proquest.com. Accessed July 24, 2015.
11. American Physical Therapy Association. PTNow website. www.ptnow.org. Accessed July 24, 2015.
12. EBSCOhost. SPORTDiscus database. www.ebscohost.com. Accessed July 24, 2015.

Chapter 12

Locating the Evidence: Search Strategies

Chapter at a Glance

Learning Outcomes

After reading this chapter, the reader will be able to:

· Define terminology related to performing a search of the literature.
· Discuss strategies for determining the best search terms.
· Describe the function of the most commonly used Boolean operators and other search parameters.
· Explain how to broaden, narrow, or limit a search.
· Outline the process for conducting a search based on a clinical question in the PICO format.

Key Terms

· Boolean operators:
  · AND
  · OR
  · NOT
  · *
· Key words
· MeSH headings

◘ FOOD FOR THOUGHT

You are a physical therapist assistant working in a skilled nursing facility and have been treating a 67-year-old woman with a diagnosis of multiple sclerosis. She experienced an exacerbation of her symptoms a couple of months ago and has been confined to bed and wheelchair since that time. However, she has been demonstrating improved overall strength and endurance during the past week, and she was able to stand in the parallel bars briefly during one of her treatment sessions this week. She has a strong desire to be able to walk again, even if she is only able to ambulate with a walker and assistance. You are interested in searching the literature to find the most effective treatment interventions for a patient with her diagnosis and at her age.

Questions to consider:

· Do you think you would have difficulty finding articles that would be helpful?

· What type of clinical question would you ask?

Introduction

In this chapter, we will complete step 2 of the evidence based practice process by discussing search strategies (Fig. 12.1). The final component is identifying appropriate search strategies to conduct the most effective search. This chapter will introduce terminology that you might encounter during a search, as well as strategies for limiting or broadening a search. Methods for tracking your search terms and strategies will also be discussed.

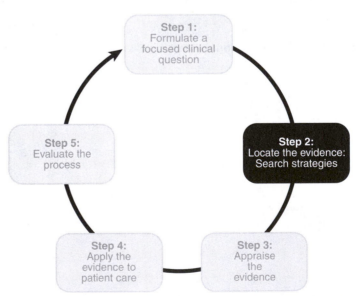

Figure 12.1 The second step of the Evidence Based Practice Process is locating the evidence. The clinician should be familiar with the most effective search strategies to efficiently locate the best evidence.

Search Terminology

The first step in beginning a search is to identify the search terms that you will use. Search terms would be selected from the clinical question. The search tool will use your search terms to match to key words in articles. **Key words** are defined as reference words that indicate the contents of a document. Authors are typically required to select key words about their article that will be utilized by search engines. Key words may be identified at the end of the abstract or elsewhere in the article. As an example, an article was published in 2010 in *Osteoarthritis and Cartilage* titled, "Does Land-Based Exercise Reduce Pain and Disability Associated With Hip Osteoarthritis? A Meta-Analysis of Randomized Controlled Trials."[1] The key words identified in the abstract are osteoarthritis, hip, exercise, randomized controlled trial, and meta-analysis. The authors identified words that would lead someone to their article if the search included any of those key words. If you had a clinical question about which exercises would be best for a patient with hip osteoarthritis, you might have entered the search terms exercise, hip, and osteoarthritis. Those search terms would have included this article in the results. Table 12.1 provides additional examples of key words from articles.

The National Institute of Medicine uses a specific list of medical terms, called medical subject headings, or **MeSH** (Fig. 12.2).[2] The list of MeSH terms was developed to streamline the storage and retrieval of published articles by providing consistent

Table 12.1 | Examples of Articles With a List of Key Words Selected by the Authors

Article Title	Key Words
"The Effect of Additional Ankle and Midfoot Mobilizations on Plantar Fasciitis: A Randomized Controlled Trial" (*Journal of Orthopedic and Sports Physical Therapy*, March 2015)	Ankle joint, dorsiflexion, joint mobilizations, plantar fascia
"Selective Recruitment of the Thoracic Erector Spinae During Prone Trunk Extension Exercise" (*Journal of Back and Musculoskeletal Rehabilitation*, March 2015)	Electromyography, thoracic extensor muscles, thoracic spine
"Improving Motor Control in Walking: A Randomized Controlled Trial in Older Adults With Subclinical Walking Difficulty" (*Archives of Physical Medicine and Rehabilitation*, November 2014)	Aging, exercise, gait, motor control, rehabilitation
"Comparative Effects of Light or Heavy Resistance Power Training for Improving Lower Extremity Power and Physical Performance in Mobility-Limited Older Adults" (*Journal of Gerontology*, March 2015)	Mobility limitations, exercise interventions, high-velocity resistance training, muscle power
"Comparison of the Effects of Water- and Land-Based Exercises on the Physical Function and Quality of Life in Community-Dwelling Elderly People With History of Falling: A Single-Blind Randomized Controlled Trial" (*Archives of Gerontology and Geriatrics*, November 2014)	Community-dwelling elderly, fear of falling, land-based exercises, physical functions, quality of life, water-based exercises

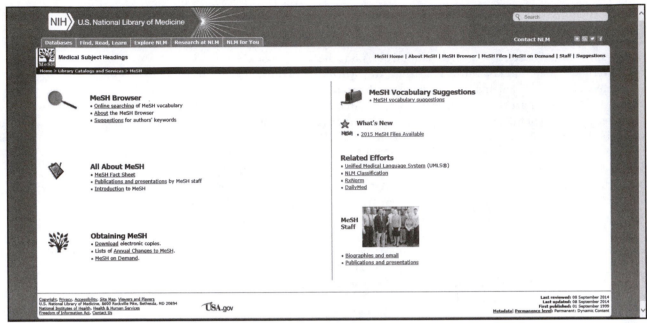

Figure 12.2 The U.S. National Library of Medicine provides resources related to medical subject headings on its website (see screenshot). The website can be accessed at http://www.nlm.nih.gov/mesh/

terminology across a large database. MeSH terms are used in MEDLINE and Index Medicus. The article on hip osteoarthritis was found using MEDLINE, so a list of MeSH terms was identified. The MeSH terms included:

- Exercise Therapy/*methods
- Osteoarthritis, Hip/*complications
- Osteoarthritis, Hip/*therapy
- Pain/*prevention & control
- Humans; Pain/etiology; Randomized Controlled Trials as Topic

As you can see, the MeSH terms are more specific than the key words. Clinicians may find the MeSH terminology more difficult to use, but it can be helpful when you want to limit your search to a very specific topic. In many instances, using search terms and key words will meet the clinician's needs.

Clinicians will often want to use more than one search term, so the search terms will need to be combined in some way. Terms can be combined using special types of words or symbols called Boolean operators. **Boolean operators** are defined as words, symbols, or phrases that will focus a search and get results that are most relevant to your question.[3,4] Let's look at how these operators can make a difference in a search. A clinician who wanted to find out which exercises would be best for a patient with hip osteoarthritis might decide to use the words "hip" and "osteoarthritis" as search terms. What would be the best way to combine the words? Is the clinician interested in articles that include both terms? If so, the terms "hip" and "osteoarthritis" would be combined with the operator **AND**. This would locate articles that included both "hip" and "osteoarthritis." Using the operator AND will narrow a search by only retrieving records that contain both words. What if the clinician wanted to locate articles that used either word? In that case, the terms "hip" and "osteoarthritis" would be combined with the operator **OR**. This would locate articles that included either "hip" or "osteoarthritis." Using the operator OR will broaden a search by retrieving records that contain either word. With the search using the operator OR, the clinician might end up with articles that dealt with knee, ankle, or back osteoarthritis. Results would also include articles about other types of hip problems besides arthritis. Figure 12.3 demonstrates the difference between AND and OR using Venn diagrams. There may be instances when you want to use OR, such as when two terms are similar but not always used together. Consider the terms "manual therapy" and "mobilization." If you were interested in articles on mobilization, you might want to enter "manual therapy" OR "mobilization" to broaden the search. To search for an exact phrase, quotation marks should be used to enclose the phrase. Quotation marks are not necessary for single or separate words.

The operator AND is the default in many search engines and databases, so if you don't type in an operator, AND will be assumed. However, that is not always the case; some search tools may default to OR. The clinician should become familiar with the search engines being used. Some search engines and databases will list the operator next to the text box for entering search terms. A drop-down menu may be available to change the operator if needed. If the operator is not listed on the search page, a summary of the search terms should be listed after a search has been conducted. The summary will list the search terms used as well as the operators used. Figure 12.4 shows the search details from a PubMed search when the terms "osteoarthritis" "back" "pain" were entered.

A number of search operators are available, but most clinicians will only use a few (Table 12.2). Two additional operators that might be useful are **NOT** and *. Use of the operator NOT narrows a search by retrieving records that do not contain the term following the operator. For example, a clinician may want to search for treatments for neck pain that do not include traction. The search terms would be entered as "neck pain" NOT traction. This would result in articles that included the exact term neck pain, but the search would exclude any articles that included the key word traction. Another operator that can be useful is the *. An asterisk will serve as a placeholder for an unknown word or when a clinician wants to allow different options for a certain word. As an example, a clinician may want to search for articles that address various mobilization methods, such as joint mobilization or spine mobilization. The clinician could enter the search terms as * mobilization. The results would likely include articles that addressed peripheral joint mobilization, soft tissue mobilization, spine mobilization, and nerve mobilization.

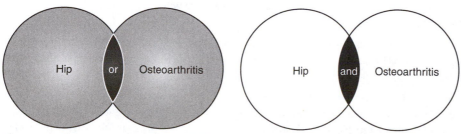

Figure 12.3 Search results using "OR" and "AND" Boolean operators. A search using the "OR" operator will locate all articles that include either word, so the search is broadened. A search using the "AND" operator will locate only those articles that include both words, so the search is narrowed.

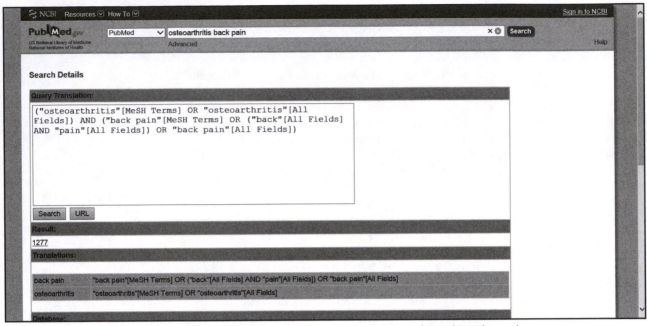

Figure 12.4 The search terms "osteoarthritis back pain" were entered into the PubMed search bar without including any operators. Pictured is a screenshot of the search details. The website was accessed at http://www.ncbi.nlm.nih.gov/pubmed/.

Table 12.2 | Examples of Search Operators

Operator	Function
" "	Quotation marks require words to be searched as a phrase in the exact order in which they are entered between the quotation marks. *Example:* to search for hip replacement as a phrase, use quotation marks—"hip replacement"
NOT or minus sign	The operator NOT or a minus sign may be used to exclude specific words from a search. *Example:* to search for neck pain but exclude items with traction, use "neck pain" NOT traction or "neck pain" – traction
OR	The operator "OR" will search for items that include either the word entered before or the word entered after the operator. *Example:* hip OR osteoarthritis will locate items that include either hip or osteoarthritis
AND	The operator "AND" will locate items that include both the word entered before and the word entered after the operator. Example: hip AND fracture will locate items that include both words hip and fracture
AND NOT	The operator "AND NOT" excludes articles containing the word(s) that follow the operator. Example: hip AND NOT fracture will locate items that include hip and will then eliminate all items that include the word fracture
NEAR	The operator "NEAR" will search for items that include both the word entered before and the word entered after the operator, with the additional requirement that the words are in close proximity to each other. Example: hip NEAR fracture will locate items that include both words within a specific proximity of each other (i.e., within 10 words).
( )	Parentheses can be used around words and operators to group them together; this requires the information within the parentheses to be processed first. Example: (hip NEAR fracture) AND replacement

The order in which items are entered can make a difference in search results. A search engine or database will typically process the terms entered from left to right, so the words entered first will be searched for first. However, Boolean operators will be treated differently. The search engine will generally process all Boolean operators AND before processing OR. You can change the order of a search by using parentheses to group certain terms together. The search engine will process information contained in parentheses first. The information below will walk the reader through an example.

A clinician wants to conduct a search about constraint-induced movement therapy (CIMT). This technique is sometimes used with patients following a stroke. The clinician recognizes that different terminology is often used for stroke, such as "CVA" or "hemiplegia." The searcher could enter the terms into the search field in a variety of ways with different results. Table 12.3 provides examples of results using MEDLINE when the terms are entered in a different order and using different operators. The first four examples show how the order of the terms can make a difference. Because a search engine processes the operator AND first, the terms that were joined by the operator AND were searched first, followed by the terms joined by the operator OR. As you can see, when the search

Table 12.3 | Search Results From MEDLINE Using Different Terms for Stroke Combined With Constraint-Induced Movement Therapy, or CIMT

Search Terms	Results
Different Order of Terms, No Grouping	
Stroke OR CVA OR hemiplegia AND constraint-induced movement therapy	**188,991 results**—included all results containing both hemiplegia and CIMT, plus all results containing stroke, plus all results containing CVA
Hemiplegia OR stroke OR CVA AND constraint-induced movement therapy	**198,154 results**—included all results containing both CVA and CIMT, plus all results containing hemiplegia, plus all results containing stroke
CVA OR hemiplegia OR stroke AND constraint-induced movement therapy	**15,494 results**—included all results containing both stroke and CIMT, plus all results containing CVA, plus all results containing hemiplegia
Separate Searches for Each Stroke Term With CITM	
Stroke AND constraint-induced movement therapy	**298 results**—results containing both stroke and CIMT
CVA AND constraint-induced movement therapy	**3 results**—results containing both CVA and CIMT
Hemiplegia AND constraint-induced movement therapy	**101 results**—results containing both hemiplegia and CIMT
Combined Search With Grouping	
(Stroke OR CVA OR hemiplegia) AND "constraint-induced movement therapy"	**363 results**—results containing any of the first three terms narrowed to those containing any of the first three terms with CIMT

terms are not grouped or ordered appropriately, the search can result in too many articles to be useful. To avoid that problem, some clinicians might choose to search for CIMT and each of the terms for stroke separately. The next three examples in Table 12.3 show the results. Clearly these searches provided much more manageable results, but this would require more time on the part of the clinician to enter several different searches. If the clinician had decided to save time and only search for "stroke" and "CIMT," articles that used "CVA" or "hemiplegia" as key words would have been overlooked. The most efficient search is one that uses a combination of Boolean operators and the appropriate placement of parentheses for grouping terms. Looking at the last example in Table 12.3, the three different terms for stroke are joined with the operator OR and enclosed in parentheses. This will force the search engine to search for all articles including any of those three terms and then to use those results to combine with the last term, "CIMT." Although 363 results may seem like a large number, the clinician should be able to scan through the titles and abstracts to narrow down the results.

Broadening, Narrowing, and Limiting a Search

There will be times when your objective will be to broaden a search. If your initial search only turned up a few results, you might want to use the Boolean operator OR and add another term. This is particularly effective when there are multiple common terms with similar meanings, as we saw with the different terms for stroke. Another strategy would be to review key terms to see if your search terms are too specific. You might also include additional databases in your search to possibly find articles in journals that are not indexed as frequently.

There will be times when you conduct a search and you come up with a list of too many results to be useful. Several strategies can be used to narrow your search. We have already seen that you could use the Boolean operator AND to combine terms during a search. The more terms you combine with AND, the more restrictive your search will be, so you need to use some caution. You might start with one or two terms, then add additional terms one at a time and see what happens to the results. Another strategy would be to review your key words to see if there might be a more specific term that could be used. For example, searching for back pain and exercise would likely yield a vast number of results. A search for back pain and extension exercises would be a little more specific, whereas a search for back pain and lumbar extension exercises would be very specific. Another strategy for narrowing your search would be to use a search engine or database that is more specific to physical therapy.

Most search engines will provide options for limiting your search. You can select a limit for the years of publication if you want to limit your results to articles published in the past 5 years or the past 10 years. Your search can be limited to peer-reviewed journals only, or you can limit your results based on the type of article (e.g., clinical practice guidelines, randomized controlled trials). You can limit your search to results with full-text only; this will eliminate results that only have the abstract or citation available. You can also limit your search to results published in English only. Keep in mind that any limit you set on your search might significantly restrict your results.

The Search Process

Now we will walk through the process of searching the literature based on a clinical question in the PICO format. We will go back to one of the scenarios from an earlier chapter:

You are working in an outpatient therapy clinic that focuses on the geriatric ortho-pedic population. The majority of patients treated at the clinic have undergone total joint replacements, such as total knees, total hips, and total shoulders. The therapist that you are teamed with has just evaluated a 64-year-old patient who underwent a total ankle replacement 3 weeks ago. The therapist has asked you to place this patient on your schedule for his next appointment. You want to become familiar with exercises that are appropriate for patients following this procedure to improve ankle function.

A clinical question based on the PICO format could be: "For geriatric patients following total ankle replacement, are therapeutic exercises effective for improving function?"

The steps below outline a method of selecting the search terms.[5] Remember that, as a clinician, you are responsible for determining your clinical question and selecting search terms. When it comes to selecting and prioritizing search terms, individual clinicians may select different search terms and may prioritize terms differently.

Step 1: Choose search terms from the PICO question. Select the terms that describe the information you want to find.
- Geriatric
- Total ankle replacement
- Therapeutic exercise
- Function

Step 2: Prioritize the search terms. This step will help you determine which terms are most important to your search; think about which terms are most likely to result in articles that are relevant to your clinical question.
- Total ankle replacement
- Therapeutic exercise
- Function
- Geriatric

Step 3: Optional: Check the MeSH terms in MEDLINE to see if your terms are the most appropriate. "Therapeutic exercise" is listed as "exercise therapy" and "function" is listed as "recovery of function."
- Replace therapeutic exercise with exercise therapy
- Replace function with recovery of function

Step 4: Finalize your list of search terms.
- Total ankle replacement
- Exercise therapy
- Recovery of function
- Geriatric

We will be using MEDLINE and CINAHL for the search. As we discussed earlier, you have a number of options for conducting a search. Let's see what happens if we search for each term individually (Table 12.4). As you can see from the results, the searches identified far too many articles to review. So let's combine some of the terms and see what happens (Table 12.5). You will notice that combining all of the terms in one search, using Boolean operators and parentheses, resulted in the same number of articles as combining total ankle replacement with each of the other terms one at a time. As you become more experienced at searching the literature, you will become more comfortable with combining terms to make your searches quicker and more efficient.

What would happen if we changed some of the parameters of our search? First, we will search another database—ProQuest (Table 12.6). The ProQuest search provided 32 results for the combined search compared with 25 results with MEDLINE and CINAHL. The difference in numbers is due to the differences in journals that are indexed by each of the search tools. Now, let's see what happens if we limit our combined search to the past 10 years (Table 12.7).

Table 12.4 | Individual Search Results

Search Terms	Results
Total ankle replacement	574 results
Exercise therapy	26,788 results
Recovery of function	32,296 results
Geriatric	95,101 results

Table 12.5 | Combined Search Results

Search Terms	Results
Total ankle replacement AND exercise therapy	2 results
Total ankle replacement AND recovery of function	23 results
Total ankle replacement AND geriatric	0 results
Total ankle replacement AND (exercise therapy OR recovery of function OR geriatric)	25 results

Table 12.6 | ProQuest Search Results

Search Terms	MEDLINE/CINAHL Results	ProQuest Results
Total ankle replacement	574 results	324 results
Exercise therapy	26,788 results	4,777 results
Recovery of function	32,296 results	5,804 results
Geriatric	95,101 results	56,306 results
Total ankle replacement AND (exercise therapy OR recovery of function OR geriatric)	25 results	32 results

Table 12.7 | Combined Search for 10 years

Search Terms: Search Limited to Last 10 Years	MEDLINE/CINAHL Results	ProQuest Results
Total ankle replacement AND (exercise therapy OR recovery of function OR geriatric)	22 results	25 results

If you compare the results of this search to the previous search, you can see that the 10-year limitation reduced some of the results more than others. However, the combined search was not reduced significantly. This indicates that most of the articles that are related to our search terms have been published in the past 10 years.

Using search terms combined appropriately with operators and parentheses, as well as limiting the search to the past 10 years, appears to have resulted in a satisfactory number of results. The search was focused enough to address the clinical question without resulting in a vast number of results to review.

Learning Task

Select a case scenario from this textbook and write a clinical question. Select search terms from your clinical question, then select a search engine or database. Enter your search terms as follows:

• Enter each search term one at a time and see how many results you get.
• Combine two of your search terms using the operator AND, then combine the same two search terms using the operator OR. Compare the results.
• Combine all of your search terms in one search using the appropriate operators and parentheses as necessary.
  • How many results did you get in the last search?
  • Was the number of results adequate for your search?

Search History

An important tool in a literature search is the search history. Most search tools will provide a search history, which provides a detailed listing of your current searches. It is helpful to locate the search history tool as you begin your searches. Although each search engine or database's search history may look different, they will all generally contain the same information. Table 12.8 provides an example of a search history for the searches we conducted previously in the MEDLINE/CINAHL databases. The search history can be helpful to review which search terms you have entered or which limits you have set. The search history is helpful for keeping track of which terms or combinations of terms have already been searched.

Table 12.8 | Search Results for the Searches Related to Total Ankle Replacement

Search #	Search Terms	Search Options	Results
9	Total ankle replacement AND (exercise therapy OR recovery of function OR geriatric)	Limiters: past 10 years Search modes: Boolean/phrase	22 results
8	Total ankle replacement AND (exercise therapy OR recovery of function OR geriatric)	Search modes: Boolean/phrase	25 results
7	Total ankle replacement AND geriatric	Search modes: Boolean/phrase	0 results
6	Total ankle replacement AND recovery of function	Search modes: Boolean/phrase	23 results
5	Total ankle replacement AND exercise therapy	Search modes: Boolean/phrase	2 results
4	Geriatric	Search modes: Boolean/phrase	95,101 results
3	Recovery of function	Search modes: Boolean/phrase	32,296 results
2	Exercise therapy	Search modes: Boolean/phrase	26,788 results
1	Total ankle replacement	Search modes: Boolean/phrase	574 results

SUMMARY

This chapter described how to conduct a literature search by using search terms and specific strategies. Search terms that most accurately reflect the information you are seeking should be selected from the clinical question. The search terms will be matched to key words in published articles to obtain search results. MEDLINE and PubMed use medical subject headings, or MeSH, to provide a common language for indexed published articles. Boolean operators, such as AND and OR, define a search's parameters and determine the order in which terms are searched. Specific strategies can be used to broaden, narrow, or limit a search. A search history will help the clinician keep track of searches for future reference.

● Case Scenario

You have been asked by a therapist in your home health facility to begin treating a new patient next week. The patient is a 57-year-old male who was involved in a motor vehicle accident 3 weeks ago. He sustained a comminuted distal tibia/fibula fracture of the right lower extremity, which was stabilized with an external fixator. He also sustained a non-displaced distal femoral fracture of the left lower extremity and is now status–post open reduction and internal fixation. He is using a wheelchair for mobility within his home. The patient is concerned because he is not able to dorsiflex or evert his right ankle, and he can barely lift his toes. The therapist is concerned about possible nerve injury caused by the comminuted fracture, but assessment was difficult due to the large amount of swelling. You would like to search the literature to determine which treatment interventions would be most effective in decreasing the edema in the patient's lower extremity with the external fixator. Write a clinical question based on the scenario and answer the following questions.

CASE QUESTIONS

1. What search terms would you use during your search?

_____

_____

2. Which of the search terms would be the most important?

_____

_____

3. How would you enter the search terms into a search engine for the most efficient search?

_____

_____

Learning Task
Using any search tool, conduct a search for the scenario described above combining your search terms in a variety of ways. What combination of search terms resulted in the most efficient search?

Review Activities

1. Explain the difference between key words and search terms.

_____

_____

_____

_____

2. Name two Boolean operators and explain the purpose of each.

_____

_____

_____

_____

3. Describe three ways to broaden a search.

_____

_____

_____

_____

4. Describe three ways to narrow a search.

_____

_____

_____

_____

5. What are MeSH headings?

_____

_____

_____

_____

MATCHING

_____ 1. AND   A. operator that broadens a search

_____ 2. Key words   B. terms developed to streamline retrieval of
                               articles

_____ 3. Boolean operators C. operator that will search for first term and
                               then eliminate results including other terms

181

_____ 4. NOT   D. words that reference document contents

_____ 5. OR   E. words, symbols, phrases to focus a search

_____ 6. MeSH headings   F. operator that narrows a search

■ References

1. Fransen M, McConnell S, Hernandez-Molina G, Reichenbach S. (2010). Does land-based exercise reduce pain and disability associated with hip osteoarthritis? A meta-analysis of randomized controlled trials. *Osteoarthritis Cartilage.* 2010;18:613-620.
2. National Institutes of Health National Library of Medicine. Medical subject headings. https://www.nlm.nih.gov/mesh/. Accessed July 25, 2015.
3. Google Websearch. Filter your search results. https://support.google.com/websearch. Accessed July 25, 2015.
4. Berkeley University Library. Basic search tips and advanced Boolean explained. http://lib.berkeley.edu/TeachingLib/Guides/Internet/Boolean.pdf. Accessed July 25, 2015.
5. Fetters L, Tilson J. *Evidence Based Physical Therapy.* Philadelphia, PA: FA Davis; 2012.

Chapter 13

Critically Appraising the Evidence

Chapter at a Glance

Learning Outcomes

After reading this chapter, the reader will be able to:

- Identify key components of a research article that are relevant to a clinical question.
- Describe the purpose of an abstract in a research article.
- Discuss key questions for critically appraising a research article related to interventions.
- Read a research article in an informed and appraising manner.

Key Terms

· Descriptive statistics
· Inferential statistics
· Minimal clinically important difference (MCID)
· Sensitivity
· Specificity

◘ FOOD FOR THOUGHT

The physical therapy department at the hospital where you just started working hosts a monthly Journal Club. You decide that it would be a good learning experience to attend. You find out the name of the article that will be discussed at the next meeting and decide to read it ahead of time. You are able to locate the article through PubMed and print a copy. The article describes an interventional study comparing iontophoresis administration of nonsteroidal anti-inflammatory medication (NSAIDs) for hamstring tendonitis to oral administration of NSAIDs. Questions to consider:
· Where would you be able to find a quick summary of the study?
· Do you think this article would be relevant to physical therapy?
· What specifics do you need to consider in order to critically appraise the article?

Introduction

Step 3 of the evidence based practice process involves critically appraising the literature located during a search (Fig. 13.1). Critically appraising the evidence begins with reviewing the search results and determining which of the articles will be useful. Reviewing the article titles should provide a good indication of the contents. A clinician may be

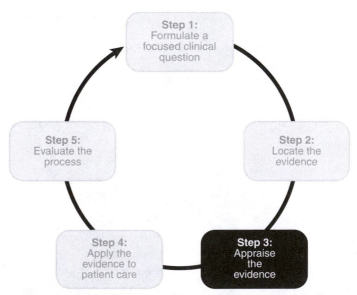

Figure 13.1 Step 3 in the Evidence Based Practice Process is critically appraising the evidence.

able to eliminate some results based simply on the title. A title, however, is limited in how much information it can provide. After reviewing titles, the next step will be to review the abstract to determine whether your time will be well spent reading the entire article. An abstract is a summary of a research article, usually limited to a specified number of words, which should allow a reader to quickly determine a paper's purpose. If the abstract makes it clear that the article is not really relevant to your clinical question, then there is no need to read the article. However, if the abstract indicates that the article is relevant to your clinical question, you will want to review the full article. In this chapter, we will discuss strategies for reviewing different types of articles. A well-written abstract will provide a concise overview of an article that includes key aspects of the study. An article should also be a concise but thorough overview of the study and study results, as well as the author's discussion and conclusions.

Appraisal Questions

The following general questions will be helpful in understanding and appraising an article (Box 13.1).[1-4] The list of results from a search will likely include different types of articles, such as research reports, case studies, diagnostic studies, narrative reviews, and systematic reviews. Every question listed here may not be appropriate for every type of article. The primary focus will be on reviewing articles related to interventions because that is the primary type of article that will be useful to the physical therapist assistant (PTA) clinician.

Box 13.1 | Questions to Help the Clinician Critically Appraise an Article

---

Appraisal Questions for Intervention Studies
1. What is the purpose of the study and is it relevant to the clinical question?
2. What types of subjects were included and are they similar to my patient?
3. Were the participants in the study randomly assigned to groups?
4. Were the groups similar at the beginning of the study?
5. Did all participants complete the study? If not, did the authors explain the reasons for noncompletion?
6. Did the study utilize blinding?
7. Did all groups in the study receive reasonable interventions and were the groups treated the same?
8. Were the treatments administered consistently?
9. Were the outcome measures appropriate for the study and do they relate to the clinical question?
10. Did the report include both descriptive and inferential statistics?
11. Did the study identify a clinically important treatment effect from the intervention?

Additional Questions for Diagnostic Studies
12. Did the study include a wide range of participants that would have included my patient?
13. Did the study make a comparison to a reference standard? If so, did all of the subjects receive both tests?
14. Did the article provide useful statistics, such as sensitivity and specificity, of the diagnostic test?

What Is the Purpose of the Study and Is It Relevant to the Clinical Question?

You should be able to determine the purpose of a study or an article easily because it should be clearly stated. The purpose should be presented in the abstract and within the first few sentences of the article, or at least within the first section of the paper. Some articles will clearly state, "The purpose of this study was . . . ." Other articles will not use such a clear statement, but the purpose should still be readily identifiable. After you determine the purpose of the study, you will need to decide if it is relevant to your question. If so, continue reading. If not, you should move on to the next article.

What Types of Subjects Were Included and Are They Similar to My Patient?

The article should provide a description of the subjects included in the study. This information should be summarized in the abstract and fully described in the Methods section of the article. In addition to a description, the inclusion and exclusion criteria should be outlined, if such criteria were used. You can also find descriptive characteristics of the subjects in the Results section of the article. Ideally you can determine whether the article is relevant by determining whether your patient would have been included in the study. However, you may have difficulty finding a study for which your patient would have qualified if there is limited research addressing the topic of your question. For example, if your question has to do with a commonly used intervention technique, you may find a large number of articles. This increases the likelihood that you would find a study for which your patient might have qualified. If your question has to do with a relatively new technique, piece of equipment, or method, or your patient is in an age category that is not as commonly studied, finding a study that might have included your patient is difficult. If your patient differs from the subjects in the study, you will need to make a decision about whether the information from the study might still be useful.

Were the Participants in the Study Randomly Assigned to Groups?

The abstract should indicate whether random assignment was used, and the Methods section should describe the assignment to groups. Random assignment is important because it can eliminate a potential source of bias and make it more likely that the groups were equal. If participants were not randomly assigned, the authors should include an explanation of why this did not occur. There are valid reasons that subjects may not have been randomly assigned, such as in studies that do not include comparison groups. Randomized controlled trials, by definition, would always include random assignment. Information about how subjects are assigned to groups will be found in the Methods section of the article. If participants could have been randomly assigned to groups but were not, the clinician must consider how important this will be in considering the results of the study and potential bias.

Were the Groups Similar at the Beginning of the Study?

This question is related to the previous question to some extent. If the participants were randomly assigned to groups, it is more likely that the groups will be similar at the beginning of the study, with a large enough number of participants. How do you determine whether the groups were similar at the beginning of the study? The Results section of the article should provide descriptive characteristics of the groups. You can review this information to determine whether the groups were similar in important characteristics and to see whether they were similar to your patient. This question is important to appraising the results of the study. If the groups were not similar at the beginning of the study, the differences at the end of the study can't be attributed to the intervention.

Did All Participants Complete the Study? If Not, Did the Authors Explain the Reasons for Noncompletion?

This information can be found under the Methods or Results sections of the article. At least 80% or more of participants should complete a study.[5] If participants drop out, the reasons for noncompletion should be addressed. A study with a high percentage of participants who do not complete the study likely had issues with the research design. If the study started with a small number of participants, losing even one or two can have a large effect on results.

Did the Study Utilize Blinding?

As discussed in previous chapters, blinding is important in reducing bias. Blinding may be applied to the evaluator, the participants, or the treating therapists. This should be clearly described in the Methods section of the article and may be included in the abstract as well. If blinding was not utilized, there should be a clear explanation of the rationale. The clinician will need to decide if this is an important factor when determining whether the results of the study are useful in answering the clinical question.

Did All Groups in the Study Receive Reasonable Interventions and Were the Groups Treated the Same?

The interventions received by each group should be described in the abstract and in the Methods section of the article. The clinician should consider whether the interventions were reasonable for comparison. The clinician also needs to consider whether the groups were treated equally. If a placebo was used, was it a reasonable placebo? If the clinician determines that it would have been obvious to participants that they were receiving the placebo, the clinician may decide not to use the study in answering the clinical question.

Were the Treatments Administered Consistently?

Investigators often have other individuals administer the treatment being studied. This may be related to blinding or to a number of other factors. An article should describe in the Methods section the treating individuals' expertise and how they were trained. The article should also describe the level of monitoring of those treatments to ensure that treatments remain consistent over time. If the patients completed treatments on their own, the type of monitoring to ensure compliance should be described.

Were the Outcome Measures Appropriate for the Study and Do They Relate to the Clinical Question?

The outcome measures should be described in the Methods section along with an explanation of why the measures were chosen. The selection of outcome measures is an important component of the research design. If the purpose of the study was to investigate the effect of an intervention on a patient's function and the only outcome measure is strength, does that seem reasonable? The outcome measure being utilized should be valid and reliable, and this should be explained in the article. The outcome measure should also be related to the clinical question. For example, if the clinical question has to do with balance and the study's outcome measure investigated gait, are those equivalent? Would a study related to gait be useful in answering a question related to balance? The clinician will need to determine whether the information will be useful.

Did the Report Include Both Descriptive and Inferential Statistics?

Experimental research articles should include both descriptive and inferential statistics.[5] **Descriptive statistics** are defined as the quantitative reporting of the main characteristics of a body of information. The purpose of descriptive statistics is to describe. Descriptive statistics provide a basic summary of the sample as well as the characteristics that were measured. Examples of descriptive statistics include frequency, mean, median, range, and percentiles. **Inferential statistics**, on the other hand, are defined as statistics that are used to reach conclusions about a set of data. These statistics provide a method for estimating characteristics of a population based on a sample. Inferential statistics are used to test hypotheses and provide some level of confidence in the results. Examples of inferential statistics include t-tests, which compare two means, and an analysis of variance (ANOVA), which compares more than two means.

Did the Study Identify a Clinically Important Treatment Effect From the Intervention?

The purpose of an intervention study is to determine whether the intervention results in a treatment effect. If the study is investigating a new exercise technique, the investigators will be interested in whether the new technique results in better outcomes than the standard or placebo treatment. This would be determined based on the inferential statistics described previously. A result that is statistically significant may not, in fact, be clinically important. Some studies will identify a **minimal clinically important difference (MCID).** The MCID is the smallest difference in a variable that would be considered an important change in a condition. If a treatment effect were identified, would the difference be large enough to be important to a patient? Consider a study that found that a new treatment technique group obtained an average improvement of 2 degrees of knee range of motion more than the standard treatment group. Would that be enough of an improvement to make a difference to a patient? Would it be likely to improve knee function? One commonly reported statistic that can help determine whether the treatment effect is clinically important is effect size. *Effect size* is defined as a method of quantifying the size of the difference between two groups.[5] Effect size can range from 0.0 to 1.0, and a commonly used guideline for interpreting effect size is as follows:

- Large: greater than 0.8
- Medium: between 0.5 and 0.8
- Small: between 0.2 and 0.5

Additional Questions for Diagnostic Studies

A few additional questions can be added for articles specifically addressing diagnostic studies. Several tools are available for appraising diagnostic studies, including the Quality Assessment of Diagnostic Accuracy Studies (QUADAS) and the Standards for Reporting of Diagnostic Accuracy (STARD).[6,7] The following questions are not as comprehensive as these tools but will provide the clinician with adequate information to appraise the article. When reviewing articles reporting diagnostic studies, you should consider the following questions:

Did the Study Include a Wide Range of Participants That Would Have Included My Patient?

For a diagnostic or prognostic study to be meaningful, the study should include a wide range of participants that represents the breadth of the condition being diagnosed. In addition, it is important to select a study that would likely have included your patient. As an example, let's assume that your 58-year-old patient has a diagnosis of rotator cuff tear, and the therapist is wondering whether the patient might have a labral lesion. You and the therapist have located a study investigating a new diagnostic test for a posteroinferior labral lesion that tested a total of 172 patients.[8] A review of the Results section of the article described the mean age and range of ages (mean 43, range 17 to 64 years of age), gender, and pretest diagnoses (including rotator cuff tear). This type of descriptive statistics would enable you to determine that your shoulder patient is similar to the subjects included in the study.

Did the Study Make a Comparison to a Reference Standard? If So, Did All of the Subjects Receive Both Tests?

Continuing with the diagnostic study identified previously, the new test was compared with both a standard clinical test and an arthroscopic evaluation. All of the subjects received both tests and the arthroscopic procedure. We discussed in Chapter 6 the importance of subjects receiving both tests in order to make a comparison. Blinding, which can reduce bias, is a consideration in exploratory studies as well as experimental studies. In the shoulder study, the surgeon performing the arthroscopic evaluation was blinded to the results of the other two tests.

Did the Article Provide Useful Statistics, such as Sensitivity and Specificity, of the Diagnostic Test?

A number of different statistics can be calculated in a diagnostic study, but one of the more commonly reported is the sensitivity and specificity of the test (Table 13.1).[9] **Sensitivity**, also called the true-positive rate, is defined as the proportion of individuals with a condition who were correctly identified by the test as positive. If a diagnostic test has high sensitivity, fewer individuals who actually have a condition are missed. **Specificity**, also called the true-negative rate, is defined as the proportion of individuals without the condition who were correctly identified by the test as negative. If a diagnostic test has high specificity, fewer individuals without the condition will test positive. A good diagnostic test would have a balance of high sensitivity and high specificity.

Learning Task

The previously identified study investigating a new test for a posteroinferior labral lesion of the shoulder described a new diagnostic test, the Kim Test. The research report indicated that the test had a sensitivity of 80% and a specificity of 94%. Is the test better at identifying the true-positive rate or the true-negative rate? Describe in your own words what the sensitivity and specificity of this test indicate.

Table 13.1 | Specificity and Sensitivity of a Diagnostic Test

Test	Condition	
	Present	**Absent**
Positive	A	B
	True Positive—condition is present and test shows positive	False Positive—condition is absent but test shows positive
Negative	C	D
	False Negative—condition is present but test shows negative	True Negative—condition is absent and test shows negative

Sensitivity = A/A + C
A test with high sensitivity, or SnOut (i.e., few false negatives) can be used to rule conditions out.

Specificity = D/B + D
A test with high specificity, or SpIn (i.e., few false positives) can be used to rule conditions in.

SUMMARY

In this chapter, we discussed steps critically appraising a research article. The abstract, which is a summary of a research article, should provide the reader with a quick way to determine whether the article might be relevant to the clinical question. In reviewing an article, the reader should be able to determine the purpose of the study and the basic information about subjects involved in the study. The reader should also attempt to determine whether the study incorporated mechanisms for reducing bias, such as random assignment and blinding. It is important to determine whether the interventions were reasonable and whether they were administered consistently. The reader should also consider whether the outcome measure was appropriate for the study. If a treatment effect was found, the reader will need to determine whether the effect size was large enough for the article to be useful in answering the clinical question. For diagnostic studies, additional questions should be answered. The reader should determine whether the article provides useful statistics, such as sensitivity and specificity. By reviewing an article with an effort to answer the questions provided, the reader should be able to read and understand basic research articles.

● Case Scenario

You are a PTA in a large academic medical center, and you are part of the acute cardiac team. Your facility has recently begun performing left ventricular assistive device, or LVAD, procedures. The therapy team is developing a physical therapy protocol to be implemented as soon as the patient is cleared to begin therapy. You have been asked to participate in the literature search and review. In conducting a literature search, you locate an article titled, "Changes in Cardiovascular Exercise Testing Parameters Following Continuous Flow Left Ventricular Assistive Device

Implantation and Heart Transplantation."[10] Using PubMed, locate the abstract for the article cited in the case scenario. Answer the following questions.

CASE QUESTIONS

1. Which of the questions listed in this chapter would you be able to answer from the abstract?

_____

_____

2. Do you have enough information to determine whether this article would be relevant to the clinical question?

_____

_____

3. How would you be able to locate the full text article?

_____

_____

Review Activities

1. What information should you be able to find in the Methods section of an article?

_____

_____

_____

_____

2. How would you be able to determine if groups were similar at the beginning of the study and why is this important?

_____

_____

_____

_____

3. What is the difference between descriptive and inferential statistics?

_____

_____

_____

_____

4. In your own words, explain effect size.

_____

_____

_____

_____

5. What is the difference between sensitivity and specificity?

_____

_____

_____

_____

MATCHING

_____ 1. Inferential statistics   A. Proportion of individuals without condition correctly tested negative

_____ 2. Descriptive statistics   B. Tests used to reach a conclusion

_____ 3. Effect size

C. Proportion of individuals with condition correctly tested positive

_____ 4. Sensitivity

D. Method of quantifying the difference between groups

_____ 5. Specificity

E. Reporting of characteristics of information

_____ 6. MCID

F. Smallest variable difference considered important

References

1. Fetters L, Tilson J. *Evidence Based Physical Therapy*. Philadelphia, PA: FA Davis; 2012.
2. Jewell DV. *Guide to Evidence-Based Physical Therapist Practice*. 3rd ed. Burlington, MA: Jones & Bartlett Learning; 2015.
3. Pyrczak F. *Evaluating Research in Academic Journals: A Practical Guide to Realistic Evaluation*. 4th ed. Glendale, CA: Fred Pyrczak ; 2008.
4. Centre for Evidence-Based Physiotherapy, University of Sydney. Physiotherapy evidence database. http://www.pedro.org.au. Accessed July 27, 2015.
5. Portney LG, Watkins MP. *Foundations of Clinical Research: Applications to Practice*. Upper Saddle River, NJ: Pearson Education; 2008.
6. University of Bristol. QUADAS: A quality assessment tool for diagnostic accuracy studies. http://www.bris.ac.uk/quadas. Accessed July 27, 2015.
7. STARD Initiative. Standards for the reporting of diagnostic accuracy studies. www.stard-statement.org. Accessed July 27, 2015.
8. Kim S, Park J, Jeong W, Shin S. The Kim Test: a novel test for posteroinferior labral lesion of the shoulder—a comparison to the Jerk Test. *Am J Sports Med*. 2005; 33(8):1188-1192.
9. Web Center for Social research methods. Research Methods Knowledge Base. www.socialresearchmethods.net. Accessed July 27, 2015.
10. Dunlay SM, Allison TG, Pereira NL. Changes in cardiopulmonary exercise testing parameters following continuous flow left ventricular assist device implantation and heart transplantation. *J Cardiac Failure*. 2014;20(8):548-554.

Chapter 14

Applying the Evidence to Patient Care

Chapter at a Glance

Learning Outcomes

After reading this chapter, the reader will be able to:

· Explain the importance of integrating evidence into patient care.
· Discuss factors that affect the integration of evidence into practice.
· Identify barriers to and strategies for integrating evidence into practice.
· Describe the importance of addressing health literacy.
· Discuss the application of the evidence based practice process in the clinical setting.

Key Term

· Innovation

◘ FOOD FOR THOUGHT

You are a physical therapist assistant in an acute inpatient rehabilitation facility, and you are working primarily with patients with diagnosis of stroke. One of the therapists just returned from a conference and was talking excitedly about a new and innovative treatment method for patients following a cerebrovascular accident (CVA). The therapist requested that the department purchase the piece of equipment required for the treatment method, which is very expensive. If the department decided to utilize the treatment method, it would require all therapists and assistants to attend a training course to become certified. The therapy manager has asked everyone to find as much information as possible about the treatment method and equipment so the rehabilitation team can discuss options during the next department meeting.

Questions to consider:

· Because this is a fairly new treatment method, do you think you will be able to locate research articles in the literature?

· How would you find information about the new treatment method and equipment?

· Should the therapy manager consider the cost of purchasing the equipment and getting all clinicians certified in making a decision about the treatment method?

Introduction

This chapter will focus on Steps 4 and 5 of the evidence based practice process. Step 4 is applying the evidence to patient care, which involves integrating new evidence with the clinician's knowledge and the patient's values and circumstances in day-to-day patient care. For the physical therapist assistant (PTA), this will also include working within the plan of care developed by the physical therapist (PT). Step 5 is evaluating the process to continually improve the clinician's skills in evidence based practice.

Factors That Affect Integration of Evidence Into Practice

The evidence based practice journey that we have taken is not complete until we successfully integrate the research evidence into clinical practice and day-to-day patient care (Fig. 14.1). Integrating the research evidence is not simply about implementing a new treatment intervention or using a new test or measure (Fig. 14.2). It also refers to communicating the best evidence to others, including patients, other health-care professionals, health-care administrators, and third-party payers. Integrating the evidence also refers to clinicians integrating the newly acquired knowledge into their existing body of knowledge and skills (Fig. 14.3). A number of factors may affect our ability to integrate research evidence into practice.

Dissemination of Innovation

Hack and Gwyer define **innovation** as "any change that represents a new method or practice."[1] They discuss the difficulty of disseminating innovative ideas in health care in general and physical therapy in particular. The traditional method of disseminating innovation is through submission of papers to peer-reviewed journals or as platform or poster presentations. In turn, the clinician must be able to access the information in a timely manner. Each step in the dissemination process can present challenges. Health-care

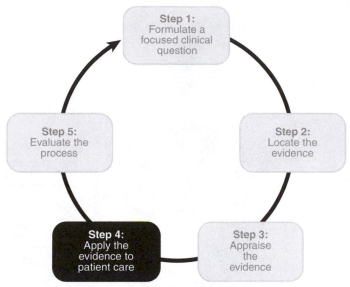

Figure 14.1 Step 4 in the Evidence Based Practice Process is applying the evidence to patient care.

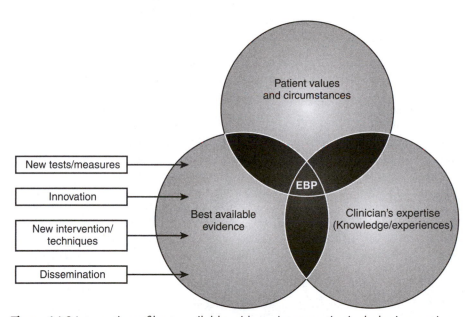

Figure 14.2 Integration of best available evidence into practice includes innovation as well as dissemination.

organizations and professional associations are making efforts to address some of these challenges by providing new and innovative means of disseminating research through the use of technology. For example, the American Physical Therapy Association (APTA) offers individuals an opportunity to attend national conferences as virtual attendees and the ability to stream lectures and presentations that have been presented at previous conferences. Professional associations are using e-mail to notify members of existing or newly developed clinical practice guidelines. Over the next few years, we will likely continue to see new methods of disseminating evidence for best practice.

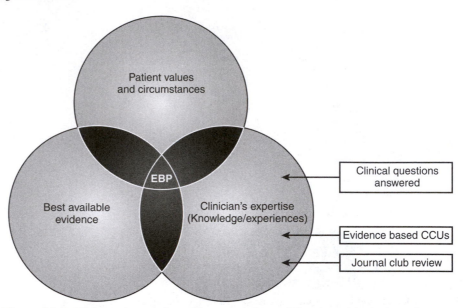

Figure 14.3 Clinicians' expertise will grow as they utiliize the evidence based process.

Clinician Acceptance

Another factor that affects the integration of evidence into practice is clinician acceptance. Clinicians are likely to accept new information, such as a new treatment technique or a new strategy for managing a particular diagnosis, if it is beneficial to their patients or their practice.[1] Clinicians are also likely to consider the cost-to-benefit ratio. Cost in this case may be price (e.g., new technology, required certification), time (e.g., time to learn, time to implement), or difficulty (e.g., difficult for patient to do or tolerate, difficult for clinicians to perform). Clinicians are more likely to accept a new technique or strategy when they perceive that the benefits outweigh the costs.

Hack and Gwyer described the patterns of adoption of innovations, or new ideas, by clinicians (Fig. 14.4).[1] Approximately 2.5% of clinicians would be categorized as "innovators" or "mavericks." These individuals are very interested in novel or unique ideas and are more likely to take risks in decision-making. An additional 13.5% would be categorized as "early adopters." This group is willing to adopt new and innovative ideas more quickly than the average clinician and tends to be more open to change. The next two categories would be "early majority" and "late majority," with each group making up 34%. The "early majority" group tends to take its lead from the "early adopters"— preferring to let others take the lead but eager to follow. The "late majority" group typically does not adopt an innovation until it is certain that the innovation is becoming accepted practice. The "laggards" or "traditionalists" make up about 16% of clinicians, and this group is most resistant to change. Someone might fall into this group who tends to say, "Why should we change? We have always done it this way."

Organizational Support

The organizational structure of a clinic or facility can play a significant role in the integration of evidence into practice.[2] An organization that focuses on best practice and evidence based practice is more likely to provide employees with the necessary resources. Resources might include continuing education opportunities; accesses to databases or journals to search for evidence; time to develop protocols, algorithms, practice patterns,

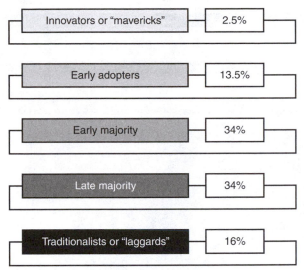

Figure 14.4 Hack and Gwyer's described patterns of adoption of innovations.

or educational materials; and organizational policies and practices, including quality improvement processes, that support innovation and best practice. Clinicians may find it more challenging to implement major changes based on evidence when an organization makes it difficult to implement change or includes multiple layers of bureaucracy.

Patient and Family Acceptance

Patient and family acceptance is another factor that affects the integration of evidence into practice. Even when a clinician is open to accepting new information, the patient, family, or both may not be as open to a new treatment technique or strategy for managing a diagnosis. Patients may prefer to continue with the current treatment rather than opting for a new treatment strategy because they do not like change. You may have heard, "When I came in for this problem before, the therapist did ..." or "I want you to do the same thing you did the last time I had this problem." Patients and families may be concerned about additional costs if the new strategy will require more visits or a longer episode of care. Or they may be resistant to a new strategy that will require fewer visits because they don't understand how they will get better with "less therapy."

A patient or family member's values and circumstances may affect the integration of evidence. Patient values are defined as the preferences that a patient or family brings to a patient care interaction. The patient's and family's preferences may be based on cultural or religious expectations, personal attitudes and beliefs, life experiences and learning, or most likely a combination of these factors. Patient circumstances are defined as the current environment or situation of the patient. This could refer to a patient's living situation, family or social situation, or resources available to provide care and manage daily living tasks.[1] Integration of best evidence must align with the patient's values and fit into the patient's circumstances in order for the patient and involved family members to be accepting.

An additional consideration is the health literacy of the patient and family members. We previously defined *health literacy* as "the degree to which individuals have the capacity to obtain, process, and understand basic health information and services needed to make appropriate health decisions."[2] The National Network of Libraries of Medicine (nnlm.gov) provides resources to address health literacy (Fig. 14.5). An

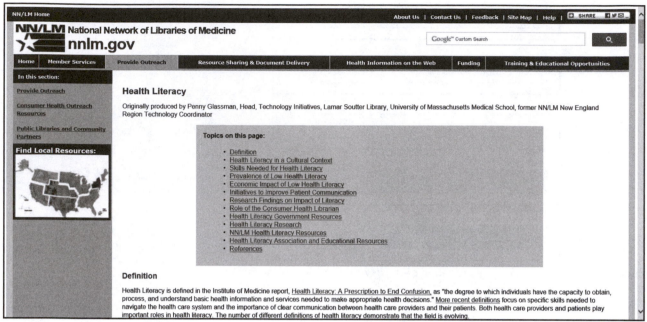

Figure 14.5 The National Network of Libraries of Medicine (www.nnlm.gov) provides resources related to Health Literacy (see screenshot). *[Screenshot source: www.nnlm.gov]*

important aspect of providing patient care is addressing a patient's health literacy through communication. For patient care to be effective, the clinician must ensure that the patient can understand explanations and instructions as well as the goals and recommendations for his or her care. Communicating physical therapy and health information to patients is very different from communicating with other health-care professionals. Clinicians need to incorporate plain language in patient communication and must ensure that they are providing unbiased information to patients and family members. Many nonprofit and professional organizations provide consumer resources that are written in a clear and concise manner. The clinician might be able to use these resources in providing additional information to a patient or family member. For example, the American Stroke Association provides updates on the organization's website of new research findings geared toward consumers. The APTA maintains a website dedicated to consumer information about physical therapy, health and prevention, and disease-specific information.

Clinician Knowledge and Skills

A clinician's existing knowledge and skills will also affect the integration of new evidence into practice. A clinician may find new evidence during a literature search that involves a treatment or diagnostic technique with which the clinician is not familiar. In that case, the clinician will not be able to incorporate the new evidence without additional training or skill acquisition. New clinicians or clinicians who are practicing in a new setting may be more likely to encounter this type of situation. In some instances, a clinician may be able to bring in a colleague who possesses the skills and knowledge necessary to incorporate best evidence into the patient's care. Otherwise, the clinician will need to choose an alternative treatment or a diagnostic technique to incorporate into the patient's care. The ethical standards of the profession include an expectation that a clinician will make clinical decisions that take into account the clinician's level of competence or expertise.

Evaluating the Process

Step 5 of the evidence based practice process is evaluating the process (Fig. 14.6). In Chapter 2, we discussed several questions that can be helpful in evaluating the process:

- Was the process helpful in answering the clinical question?
- If the process was not helpful, what might you have done differently?
- If the process was helpful, what might you do in the future to make the process more efficient or effective?
- What was the patient's outcome?

Not every search for evidence will be successful, and not every piece of evidence that you identify will be helpful in answering the clinical question. As clinicians become more experienced in evidence based practice, they will learn to quickly identify the best search tool and the best source for specific types of questions. For example, if a question is related to a medical procedure or medical treatment, a search tool that focuses on journals or articles in the field of medicine or nursing might be most useful. If a question is related to rehabilitation, the clinician may choose to use a search tool that focuses on journals or articles that address rehabilitation, physical therapy, occupational therapy, and rehabilitation nursing. The last question is important in expanding a clinician's knowledge base and experience. Not every patient will respond to an intervention in the same way, so your patient may not respond as you expected based on the evidence.

The final step, evaluating the process, may not seem as critical as the first four steps, particularly to a clinician who is pressed for time. However, clinicians who skip this step will not become as skilled or efficient in evidence based practice as they might have otherwise. Step 5 can also include sharing the evaluation of the process with other clinicians, such as providing an in-service to your colleagues to share your experience. Other clinicians will benefit from learning about your clinical question, the steps you

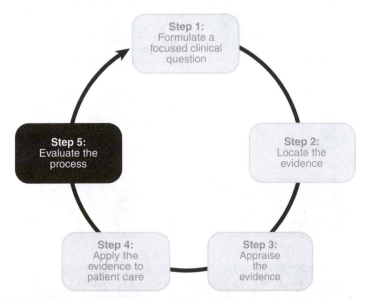

Figure 14.6 Step 5 in the Evidence Based Practice Process is evaluating the process. Evaluating the process is important in expanding a clinician's knowledge base and experience.

took to locate evidence, your appraisal of the evidence, and your patient's outcomes. You should also address any mistakes you made along the way and how you would improve the process the next time.

Putting It All Together

In this text, we have described the evidence based process as a series of five separate steps. However, a clinician may repeat the first steps multiple times during a single patient's episode of care. The clinician may have clinical questions early in the patient's care and continue to have different clinical questions throughout the patient's care. To assist the reader with understanding all steps of the evidence based practice process, we will walk through the entire process using the patient scenario below (Fig. 14.7):

You are a PTA working in a small-town practice that provides therapy in the community hospital and the outpatient clinic. You are the only PTA working with two PTs in the practice. The therapist informed you today that she just evaluated

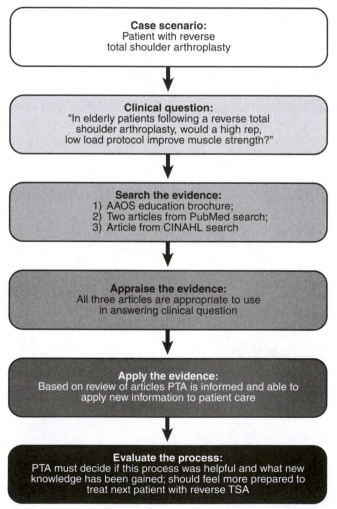

Figure 14.7 The Evidence Based Practice Process, or putting it all together.

a 72-year-old woman in the outpatient clinic. The patient had a reverse total shoulder arthroplasty 3 months ago because of a history of right shoulder post-traumatic arthritis. The therapist is going to place the patient on your schedule for tomorrow, so she provided you with the written plan of care. The goals address improving functional active range of motion, improving strength and muscle performance, and maximizing shoulder function. The therapist informed you that the patient has been cleared by the surgeon to progress from active range of motion exercises to progressive resistance exercises.

The patient lives with her daughter but spends much of the day at home alone. A granddaughter has been staying with the patient and helping her with activities of daily living, but the granddaughter is returning to college this week. The patient's primary language is Spanish, but her daughter and granddaughter are bilingual. She feels that she has been a burden to her daughter and granddaughter, so she wants to regain her independence as soon as possible.

You have treated patients who had conventional total shoulder replacements, but you have never worked with anyone following a reverse procedure. Although you have some knowledge about the procedure, you would like to find out more information about the procedure and the expected outcomes. You would also like to find out what type of exercise protocol would be best for this patient.

Step 1: Formulate a Focused Clinical Question

You begin formulating your clinical questions related to this patient. Your first clinical question, a background question, is the most general question and fairly broad. You formulate the following question:

"What does the reverse total shoulder surgery involve and what are common complications?"

Your second question is also a background question and is focused on outcomes:

"In elderly patients following a reverse total shoulder arthroplasty, what are the expected outcomes?"

Your third question is related to interventions. Based on your clinical knowledge, you decide that you should incorporate a low-load, high-repetition strengthening protocol with this patient. However, you would like to search the literature to determine whether this type of protocol will be effective for improving your patient's arm strength. You formulate the following foreground clinical question:

"In elderly patients following a reverse total shoulder arthroplasty, would a high-repetition, low-load protocol improve muscle strength?"

Step 2: Locate the Evidence

You happen to have a 30-minute gap in your schedule today because of a patient cancellation, so you decide to use that time to search for evidence. Your first thought for finding background information is to search in the reference books kept in the PT department. None of the books, however, has any information about this type of surgical procedure. You recall that you have previously found information about orthopedic surgical procedures at the American Academy of Orthopaedic Surgeons (AAOS) website (www.aaos.org), so you search for information there.[3] You type in "reverse total shoulder" and find a helpful educational handout that describes the procedure, lists some potential complications, and briefly talks about long-term outcomes. Although this is a good start, you would like more in-depth information.

For your background questions, you decide to use PubMed to search a broad range of journals that cover medicine. Because this procedure is fairly new in the United States, you decide to search broadly for any type of research article related to your search terms. For the initial search, you choose the following search terms: "reverse total shoulder" AND outcomes. The search results in 78 articles found. You scan the titles and identify two articles that you think will be most helpful in answering your questions: "Reverse Total Shoulder Arthroplasty: A Review of Results According to Etiology" and "What Is a Successful Outcome Following Reverse Total Shoulder Arthroplasty?"[4,5]

Your foreground question is related to physical therapy and rehabilitation, so you decide to add CINAHL to your search. You choose the following search terms: "reverse total shoulder" AND (exercise OR therapy OR rehabilitation). Your search results in 15 articles. You choose one article that looks as though it is most relevant to your question, which is entitled, "Rehabilitation Following Reverse Total Shoulder Arthroplasty."[6]

Step 3: Critically Appraise the Evidence

You were able to locate four pieces of evidence during your search. The information from the AAOS website is written for the public and is a broad overview of the procedure. This piece of evidence would be categorized as expert opinion or a narrative report. The first two research articles you located described longitudinal cohort studies that followed patients after a reverse total shoulder procedure for 2 to 3 years. The article addressing rehabilitation is a clinical commentary written by three PTs and an orthopedic surgeon. Although it is not a research article, it outlines a therapy protocol for patients following a reverse total shoulder arthroplasty. You critically appraise the articles using the questions from Chapter 13 of this text as a guideline. Based on your appraisal, you decide that the articles are appropriate to answer your clinical questions. You read the articles and feel well prepared to begin treating your patient tomorrow.

Step 4: Apply the Evidence to Patient Care

As you begin treating the patient, you feel informed and prepared to answer any questions that the patient may have. For example, if the patient asks about the expected level of function following this type of surgery, you should be prepared to answer the patient's questions. Even though the patient wants to become independent as soon as possible, you discuss with her the potential complications that can occur if she doesn't adhere to the precautions provided by her surgeon. Your understanding of the surgical procedure helps you understand the restrictions placed on the patient's movement by the surgeon, and you can explain these to the patient. You can also visualize the placement of the prosthetic components as you instruct the patient in proper movement of the shoulder to gradually restore mobility to the joint. You are better able to educate the patient and family about joint protection, posture, and the proper technique for performing bed mobility and transfers. You notice that the patient appears to have difficulty reading the exercise instructions. When you ask her if she understands, she tells you that although she is able to speak English fairly well, she has difficulty reading in English. You are able to reprint the exercise program in Spanish, which will help the patient understand and follow the instructions appropriately.

As you continue to work with this patient throughout her rehabilitation, you might come up with additional clinical questions. The steps in the evidence based practice process can be repeated as often as needed to address clinical questions and improve patient care.

Step 5: Evaluate the Process

After the patient has completed an episode of care, you should evaluate the entire process. You should decide whether the process was helpful in answering the clinical question or questions. In this case, you decide that the process was helpful because you were able to locate articles that provided the information you needed. Because the process was helpful, what might you do in the future to make the process more efficient or effective? Your answer to this question may be that you would conduct the search in the same way the next time. However, if you tried a number of different search strategies before you were able to identify helpful articles, you might identify the most effective strategy to use the next time. The last question to ask is about the patient's outcome. If this patient had a successful functional outcome, the evidence you used during her episode of care would be integrated into your experience and your knowledge base as being effective. If the patient did not have a successful functional outcome, that information will also become part of your experience and your knowledge base as being less than effective. The next time you treat a patient who underwent a reverse total shoulder arthroplasty, you will be more experienced and knowledgeable from the beginning. You may still encounter clinical questions, but you will be prepared to search for evidence to expand your knowledge in this area even more.

SUMMARY

PTs and PTAs work together as patient care teams and should strive together for best practice based on evidence. Factors that affect the integration of evidence into practice include dissemination of innovation, clinician acceptance, organizational support, patient and family acceptance, and clinician knowledge and skills. Clinicians should strive to improve health literacy through effective communication. Although most information related to evidence based practice is aimed at therapists, the PTA plays an important role, particularly in the patient management elements of Intervention, Tests and Measures, and Outcomes. Clinicians should be able to utilize the evidence based practice process to improve patient care and facilitate better patient outcomes. The next few years are likely to bring many more advances in health care and technology, so clinicians must be skilled in managing the ever-growing body of knowledge.

● Case Scenario

You are a PTA working in a large hospital, and you primarily see patients in the intensive care unit (ICU). You are a member of the facility's Early Mobilization Committee, which was appointed to develop policies and procedures for early mobilization with a goal of decreasing ICU and hospital length of stay. Discussion during the meeting today addressed the concern of increased falls when patients are mobilized too early. You volunteered to conduct a literature search to find evidence related to other facility's early mobilization programs and their outcomes, including whether falls were noted as an issue. You are also interested in determining the appropriate role of the PTA in an early mobilization program.

CASE QUESTIONS

1. Would you limit your search to physical therapy literature in this case? Why or why not?

_____

_____

2. Would you limit your search to randomized controlled trials and systematic reviews? Why or why not?

_____

_____

3. What other options would you consider for finding information in addition to a literature search?

_____

_____

Learning Task

Using any search tool, locate a research article about an early mobilization program in an acute care setting.

• What type of study is described in the article?
• Do the results of the study identify any benefits to the early mobilization program?
• If so, what are the benefits? What were the outcomes of the study?

Review Activities

1. List two examples of disseminating innovation.

   _____

   _____

   _____

   _____

2. In your own words, explain the difference in adoption of new ideas between the "early majority" and the "late majority."

   _____

   _____

   _____

   _____

3. Briefly explain how organizational support can affect the integration of evidence into practice.

   _____

   _____

   _____

   _____

4. Why is Step 5 of the evidence based practice process important?

   _____

   _____

   _____

   _____

MATCHING

_____ 1. Innovation   A. Therapist willingness to adopt new ideas

_____ 2. Health literacy   B. A change that represents new practice

_____ 3. Patient values   C. Patient's ability to process health information

_____ 4. Patient circumstances D. Patient and family preferences

_____ 5. Clinician acceptance E. Patient and family environment

■ References

1. Hack LM, Gwyer J. *Evidence Into Practice: Integrating Judgment, Values, and Research.* Philadelphia, PA: F. A. Davis; 2013.

2. Fetters L, Tilson J. *Evidence Based Physical Therapy.* Philadelphia, PA: FA Davis; 2012.

3. American Academy of Orthopedic Surgeons. AAOS website. www.aaos.org. Accessed July 27, 2015.

4. Wall B, Nove-Josserand L, O'Connor DP, Edwards B, Walch G. Reverse total shoulder arthroplasty: a review of results according to etiology. *J Bone Joint Surg Am.* 2007; 89(7):1476-1485.

5. Roy JS, Macdermid JC, Goel D, Faber KJ, Athwal GS, Drosdowech DS. What is a successful outcome following reverse total shoulder arthroplasty? *Open Orthop J.* 2010;4:157-163.

6. Boudreau S, Boudreau ED, Higgins LD, Wilcox RB 3rd. Rehabilitation following reverse total shoulder arthroplasty. *J Orthop Sports Phys Ther.* 2007;37(12):734-743.

Glossary

Abstract: summary of a research study, often limited to 250 words or less; usually contains the purpose of the study, brief description of methods and results, and a conclusion

Accessible population: the actual group of subjects available to be selected for the study

Active (positive) control group: control group in which the subjects receive a standard treatment rather than a placebo

Applied research: research that seeks to solve practical problems and is usually grounded in basic science research; is conducted under actual situational conditions rather than in a laboratory setting

Background question: clinical question that focuses on the typical course of a disease, an injury, or the typical management of a problem

Basic research: the study and research of science aimed at increasing scientific knowledge; is often theoretical in nature; attempts to increase the understanding of scientific phenomena without attempting to solve or treat problems

Between-subjects design: another name for independent groups design

Bias: any tendency that prevents unprejudiced consideration of a question

Blinding: method for ensuring that individuals involved in a study do not know the group assignment of the subjects

Boolean operators: words, symbols, or phrases that will focus a search and get results that are most relevant to your question
- **AND:** Boolean operator that will narrow a search by identifying only results that include both search terms joined by AND
- **OR:** Boolean operator that will broaden a search by identifying results that include either of the search terms joined by OR
- **NOT:** Boolean operator that will search for results that include the first term and then eliminate results that include the term following NOT
- ***:** an asterisk serves as a placeholder for an unknown word or when a clinician wants to allow different options for a certain word

Carryover effect: the effect of one intervention continuing into the next test period

Case-control study: a study in which subjects are selected based on whether or not they have the condition being investigated

Case report: in-depth description of a case study or case series

Cases: the subjects who have the condition being investigated

Case series: a detailed description of individual patients or clients with similar diagnoses or circumstances and their outcomes

Case study: a detailed description of an individual patient or client and the outcomes of the case

CINAHL: Cumulative Index to Nursing and Allied Health Literature; database that indexes more than 5,000 journals from nursing and other health-care disciplines, including physical therapy

Clinical decision rule: a combination of findings that have demonstrated meaningful predictability in determining a specific condition or diagnosis

Clinical practice guidelines: evidence based recommendations for the diagnosis, treatment, or prevention of health-care problems that are typically developed by a panel of experts

Clinical question: a question that provides the basis for a literature search to find information relevant to a particular patient situation

Clinical research: research involving human subjects aimed at increasing knowledge of disease or injury, diagnosis, treatment, or management of conditions

Clinician: an individual who has patient care responsibilities; in this text, the term refers to the physical therapist or the physical therapist assistant

Cochrane Collaboration: a nonprofit organization in the United Kingdom that advocates evidence based decision-making and provides a database of evidence primarily geared toward systematic reviews and meta-analyses

Cochrane Library: library that is part of the Cochrane Collaboration; maintains a number of databases that are geared toward evidence based practice in health care

Cohort: a group of subjects followed over time

Cohort study: a study that follows a specific cohort, or group, over a period of time

Comparison group: a group of subjects used for comparison to an experimental group or groups

Conference proceeding: a published version of the papers and abstracts presented at a conference

Control: designated intervention, or absence of intervention, that will be used as a comparison to the intervention of choice in a PICO question

Control group: group of subjects who will not receive the experimental intervention and are used as a comparison for the experimental group

Controls: the subjects who do not have the condition being investigated; should be matched to the cases on relevant factors such as age or gender

Correlational study: a study designed to identify the relationship, or degree of association, between variables

Crossover design: repeated measures research design in which the subjects are randomly assigned to groups and the groups complete the conditions of the study in a different order

Cross-sectional study: a study that investigates groups of subjects at one point in time and compares the characteristics of the different groups

DARE: Database of Abstracts of Reviews of Effects; database that focuses primarily on systematic reviews of the effects of health-care interventions

Database: an organized system containing lists of citations of references; may include the reference summary, the reference summary and abstract, or the full text of the article

Dependent variable: the variable being measured as an outcome

Descriptive research: research that investigates and documents variables of the population of interest; what are the characteristics of the sample and do the characteristics change over time?

Descriptive statistics: the quantitative reporting of the main characteristics of a body of information

Descriptive survey: a research method designed to gather data to describe the characteristics, behaviors, or attitudes of a particular group

Developmental research: research that describes developmental behaviors and the normal sequence and changes over time

Diagnosis: description of a patient condition obtained by evaluating the data obtained during an examination

Diagnostic test or measure: measure used to obtain objective information during the diagnostic process

Double-blind study: study in which neither the subjects nor the researcher is aware of the group assignment during the study

Effect size: a method of quantifying the size of the difference between two groups

Ethnography: the study of attitudes, beliefs, and behaviors of a culture through observation of individuals within their own setting

Etiology: cause of a disease or condition; may include a specific set of factors that contribute to the disease or condition occurrence

Evidence: the available body of scientific research literature that can be used to answer a clinical question

Evidence based medicine: the conscientious, explicit, and judicious use of current best evidence in making decisions about the care of individual patients

Evidence based practice: the integration of the best available research evidence with the clinician's expertise and the patient's individual values and circumstances

Experimental group: group of subjects who will undergo the experimental intervention

Experimental research: research that investigates a cause-and-effect relationship between variables; in other words, does the independent variable x cause a change in the dependent variable y?

Exploratory research: research that investigates relationships between variables; in other words, is a change in variable x related to a change in variable y?

Factorial design: research design that includes two or more independent variables, or factors

Filtered (secondary) source: source that contains information derived from previously published material and includes an evaluation, a review, or some other interpretation of the material

Foreground question: clinical question that focuses on making clinical decisions related to patient management.

Generalization: the ability to reasonably apply the results of a study conducted on a sample to all individuals within the population

Grounded theory: a research method that involves the discovery of theory through the analysis of data; the theory is "grounded" in the data

Health literacy: the degree to which individuals have the capacity to obtain, process, and understand basic health information and services needed to make appropriate health decisions

Independent groups design: research design in which subjects are assigned to and participate in only one group (e.g., experimental group or control group, but not both)

Independent variable: the variable being manipulated by the researcher

Inferential statistics: statistics that are used to reach conclusions about a set of data

Informed consent: the process by which the clinician discloses appropriate information to a competent patient so that the patient can make a voluntary choice to accept or refuse treatment

Innovation: any change that represents a new method or practice

Intervention: purposeful interaction of a physical therapist or physical therapist assistant with a patient using physical therapy procedures and techniques to produce change

Key words: reference words that indicate the contents of a document

Likert scale: a measurement scale designed to allow respondents to identify their level of agreement or disagreement with an item in order to capture the intensity of perceptions or feelings

Longitudinal study: a study that follows a group of subjects over time and collects data at repeated intervals

MEDLINE: biomedical database maintained by the National Library of Medicine; can be accessed through PubMed

MeSH headings: medical subjects headings; a list of terms developed to streamline the storage and retrieval of published articles by providing consistent terminology across a large database

Meta-analysis: a type of systematic review that pools the data from separate but similar experiments of different researchers and conducts a statistical analysis of the pooled data

Methodological research: research designed to develop and/or test a new measurement tool that can be used in the clinical setting

Minimal clinically important difference (MCID): smallest difference in a variable that would be considered an important change in a condition

Narrative review: report typically written by an expert in a specified field that provides an overview of a topic

Nonparametric tests: statistical tests that do not make assumptions about the population distribution or the data being collected

Nonprobability sampling: method of sampling that is not random; members of the population do not all have the same probability of being selected

Normative research: research designed to collect data in order to describe standard values of a particular characteristic of a population

No-treatment control group: control group in which the subjects receive no treatment as opposed to a placebo

One-way (single-factor) design: research design that includes only one independent variable, or factor

Outcome: change in a patient's condition as a result of an intervention

Parametric tests: statistical tests that make assumptions about the population distribution and the data being collected

Patient-centered care: a model of health care in which patients actively participate in their own health care and the patient and family are the center of care

Patient circumstances: the current environment or situation of a patient, such as a patient's living situation, family or social situation, or resources available to provide care and manage daily living tasks

Patient values: the preferences that a patient or family brings to a patient care interaction; patient's and family's preferences may be based on cultural or religious expectations, personal attitudes and beliefs, life experiences, and learning

PEDro: Physiotherapy Evidence Database; a database of abstracts of clinical trials, systematic reviews, and clinical practice guidelines related to physical therapy

Peer review: process of evaluation of an article or a similar work by individuals who are considered experts in the field in order to ensure that certain standards are met

Peer-reviewed research: studies that have been submitted for scrutiny by experts in the field who provide feedback, typically anonymous, on any or all aspects of the research; this process of critical review before publication is considered the gold standard

Phenomenology: a research method of explaining complex phenomena by analyzing narrative information provided by individual subjects and identifying themes

PICO: an acronym that can guide the clinician in developing a clinical question; the letters represent **P**atient, **I**ntervention, **C**omparison Intervention (or **C**ontrol), and **O**utcome

Placebo: a harmless medication or procedure that has no therapeutic effect and is used as a comparison to an experimental medication or procedure; the placebo group would reasonably be expected to show no improvement

Placebo control group: control group in which the subjects receive a placebo, or sham, intervention

Plain language: clear, straightforward expression that uses as few words as possible to convey a message

Population of interest: the target population; the group of individuals who meet a specific set of criteria defined in a research study

Post-test: test or measure that is conducted at the end of an intervention period

Power: the probability that a study will detect an intervention effect of a specified size that is statistically significant

Predictive study: a type of correlational study that predicts an outcome based on the relationship between variables

Pre-test: test or measure that is conducted before an intervention period

Probability sampling: sampling method that uses random selection, most likely to result in a sample that truly represents the population

Prognosis: determination of the expected functional outcome and the time frame needed to achieve the outcome

Prospective: data collection from a defined point of time and moving forward

Prospective study: an investigation that collects new data during a specified period of time

PTNow: research tool for members of the American Physical Therapy Association; includes ArticleSearch, Clinical Summaries, and Guidelines

Publication bias: the decreased likelihood of publication for research with negative or nonsignificant results compared with research with positive results

Qualitative research: research that collects non-numerical, or verbal, data through exploratory and descriptive methods; emphasizes the individual perspective by describing aspects of human nature and individuals' perception of their own experiences

Quantitative research: research that collects numerical data and utilizes statistical methods

Quasi-experimental design: experimental research design that lacks random assignment, a comparison group, or both

Random assignment: method of assigning subjects to groups such that each subject chosen for the study has an equal chance of being assigned to a specific group

Randomized controlled trial (RCT): study in which subjects are assigned randomly to groups to receive one of several interventions, of which one intervention is a control group; the purpose of an RCT is to compare the outcomes and determine whether any differences exist

Random selection: method of selection in which every individual within the population has an equal chance of being selected for the sample

Reliability: the ability to produce the same results in repeated measures when the conditions are the same

Repeated measures design: experimental research design in which each subject participates in each condition of the experiment

Research hypothesis: a statement that proposes or predicts the relationship between variables prior to a study being conducted

Research question: a question that provides the basis for a research study and is sometimes restated as a research hypothesis; must be developed in such a way that an answer can be determined using the scientific method

Research report: report of original research

Research review synopsis: brief, focused summary of a systematic review or meta-analysis that includes commentary by the professional completing the synopsis

Retrospective: data that was collected in the past, such as data from patient medical records

Retrospective study: an investigation of data that has already been collected in the past

Sample: a subset of a population that is selected for a study; should demonstrate the same characteristics and variability as the larger group

Sampling bias: the over- or under-representation of certain characteristics of the population within the sample

Search engine: an information retrieval system that searches electronic databases and other Internet resources

Sensitivity: the proportion of individuals with a condition who were correctly identified by the test as positive

Shared decision-making: a collaborative process of decision-making that allows patients and health-care providers to make health-care decisions together by taking into account the best available evidence, the provider's clinical experience, and the patient's values and preferences

Single-blind study: study in which one of the parties involved (researcher, subject) was blinded, but not the other

Specificity: is the proportion of individuals without the condition who were correctly identified by the test as negative

SPORTDiscus: comprehensive database that is focused on sports and sports medicine

Study synopsis: brief, focused summary of a study that includes commentary by the professional reviewing the study

Systematic review: a literature review that focuses on a specific research or clinical question; includes (1) identification of all relevant studies, focusing on randomized controlled trials; (2) assessment of the quality of studies identified; (3) selection of the highest quality and most relevant studies; and (4) a synthesis of the results.

Unfiltered (primary) source: source containing the first report of a study with no outside evaluation or interpretation of the report

Validity: the soundness or accuracy of a conclusion or measurement

Variable: a characteristic that can be manipulated or observed and can take on different values

Washout period: period of rest between test periods that should provide time for the effects of the first treatment to be eliminated

Within-subjects design: another name for repeated measures design

Index

Page numbers followed by "f" denote figures, "t" denote tables, and "b" denote boxes